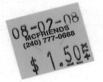
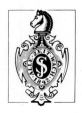

Treatment in Clinical Medicine

Series Editor: John L. Reid

Forthcoming titles in the series:

Rheumatic Disease
Hilary A. Capell, T.J. Daymond, and W. Carson Dick

The Elderly
W. MacLennan, A. Shepherd and I.H. Stevenson

Cardiovascular Disease
A.R. Lorimer and W. Stewart Hillis

Neurological and Neuro-psychiatric Disorders
J.D. Parkes, P. Jenner, D. Rushton and C.D. Marsden

Hypertension
B.N.C. Prichard and C.W.I. Owens

Respiratory Disease
Anne E. Tattersfield and M. McNicol

Gastrointestinal Disease

Edited by
C.J.C. Roberts

Springer-Verlag
Berlin Heidelberg New York Tokyo 1983

C.J.C. Roberts, MD, MRCP
Consultant Senior Lecturer in Clinical Pharmacology,
Department of Medicine,
Bristol Royal Infirmary, Bristol, England

Series Editor:
John L. Reid, MD, FRCP
Regius Professor of Materia Medica,
University of Glasgow, Scotland

ISBN 3-540-12531-0 Springer-Verlag Berlin Heidelberg New York Tokyo
ISBN 0-387-12531-0 Springer-Verlag New York Heidelberg Berlin Tokyo

Library of Congress Cataloging in Publication Data
Main entry under title:
Gastrointestinal Disease
(Treatment in clinical medicine)
Bibliography: p. Includes index.   1. Gastrointestinal
system—Diseases—Treatment—Addresses, essays, lectures. I. Roberts, C.J.C.
(Clive John Charlton), 1946–   . II. Series. [DNLM: 1. Gastrointestinal
diseases—Diagnosis. 2. Gastrointestinal diseases—Therapy. WI 100 G2586]
RC802.G37   1983   616.3   83-10442
ISBN 0-387-12531-0 (U.S.)

Typeset by Wilmaset, Birkenhead, Merseyside
Printed by Robert Hartnoll Ltd, Bodmin, Cornwall

2128/3916-543210

Series Editor's Foreword

"Gastrointestinal Disease" is the first monograph in a new series on management and treatment in major clinical subspecialties and patient groups. Further volumes will be published over the next few years. Each book is complete in its own right. The whole series, however, has been prepared to fill a gap, perceived by the publisher, myself and the volume authors, between standard textbooks of medicine and therapeutics and research reviews, symposia and original articles in specialist fields. Each volume aims to provide a concise, up to date account of treatment in its subject area with particular reference to drug therapy. Traditional clinical and therapeutic approaches have been presented in the context of developments in clinical pharmacology. Wherever possible, authorship has been undertaken by practising clinicians who themselves have training and experience in clinical pharmacology. The volumes are intended to be guides to treatment, to assist in the choice of drug and other treatment and to provide easy references to drug interactions and adverse reactions. It is expected that these monographs will be particularly useful for the young hospital doctor in training for higher qualifications. However, they should also be valuable to senior medical students and to those in established hospital or general practice who are seeking to update their knowledge and to view recent developments in other fields in a balanced context.

The aims of the series should be upheld by this volume on "Gastrointestinal Disease". The book has been prepared in Bristol, one of the acknowledged centres of Gastroenterology in Britain at present. The Editor, Dr. Clive Roberts, is not only a respected clinician but has a wide clinical and research experience in clinical pharmacology, particularly relating to the liver and the gastrointestinal tract. Dr. Roberts has assembled a distinguished list of co-authors with expertise in a range of areas of gastroenterology from the oesophagus to the colon. In addition, Dr.

Roberts writes on the important influence of gastrointestinal pathology and liver disease especially on the disposition and action of drugs given for other conditions.

This volume will be followed in the near future by volumes on "Rheumatic Disease" by H. Capell, T. Daymond and C. Dick and "The Elderly" by W. MacLennan, A. Shepherd and I.H. Stevenson. Further volumes are planned to cover Cardiovascular Disease, Respiratory Disease, Neurological and Neuro-psychiatric Disorders, and Hypertension.

Glasgow, July 1983   John L. Reid

Preface

Drug usage plays a relatively minor role in the treatment of disease of the gastrointestinal tract. Here supportive measures such as attention to nutritional needs, avoidance of substances which may cause exacerbations and use of surgical procedures assume an importance in symptomatic relief and cure at least as great as the use of pharmacological agents. Accurate diagnosis of disease entity and assessment of the effects of the disease on the body remain the cornerstone of gastroenterological practice. Once the patient's disease has been defined treatment may proceed logically and often simply. The need for accurate diagnosis of disease in inaccessible and elusive parts of the alimentary system has stimulated the development of great improvements in techniques of organ imaging and visualisation. The advances in diagnostic techniques by fibre-optic endoscopy, ultrasound and computerised axial tomography over the past few years have greatly outstripped any advances in the therapeutics of gastrointestinal disease. However, these advances have had considerable therapeutic implication for it is now possible to determine the efficacy of drug treatment more accurately. This is most apparent in the treatment of peptic ulceration, where the advent of histamine H_2 receptor antagonists coincided with the widespread availability of upper gastrointestinal endoscopy. Treatments previously had suffered the great disadvantage that their ulcer-healing power could only be assessed by often misleading barium contrast radiology. At present, old-fashioned treatments long since rejected as of only symptomatic benefit have not been scientifically evaluated by modern techniques.

The aim of this book is to provide practical guidance to the hospital physician in the management of gastrointestinal disease in the light of present knowledge. It has been written by a group of physicians with particular experience in gastroenterology. No one aspect of management has been emphasised to the neglect of others. The uses and disadvantages, indications and contra-indications of diagnostic techniques and therapeutic procedures have been discussed as fully as experience or evidence allows. Doctors should 'do no harm' and so we have made a point of mentioning common prescribing pitfalls when caring for patients with gastrointestinal disease. The format of each chapter in the book is similar for ease of reference, and there is a section containing useful information about drugs likely to be used. The book is thus intended to be sufficiently readable for the candidate studying for MRCP and sufficiently accessible for the physician faced with an immediate clinical problem.

Bristol, April 1983   C.J.C. Roberts

Contents

SECTION II

Contributors

R.E. Barry, BSc, MD, FRCP
Consultant Senior Lecturer in Medicine
Bristol Royal Infirmary

B.T. Cooper, BSc, MD, MRCP
Lecturer in Medicine
Bristol Royal Infirmary

T.K. Daneshmend, MB, MRCP
Tutor in Clinical Pharmacology
Bristol Royal Infirmary

M.J. Hall, MB, MRCP
Lecturer in Medicine
Bristol Royal Infirmary

K.W. Heaton, MA, MD, FRCP
Reader in Medicine
Bristol Royal Infirmary

M.M.A. Homeida, MD, MRCP
Consultant Lecturer in Medicine
University of Khartoum, Sudan

A.P. Manning, MD, MRCP
Senior Registrar in Medicine
Yorkshire Region

R.A. Mountford, BSc, MD, MRCP, FRCR
Consultant Senior Lecturer in Medicine
Bristol Royal Infirmary

A.E. Read, MD, FRCP
Professor of Medicine
Bristol Royal Infirmary

C.J.C. Roberts, MD, MRCP
Consultant Senior Lecturer in Clinical Pharmacology
Bristol Royal Infirmary

SECTION I

1 Oesophageal Disease

R. A. Mountford

Oesophagitis

Pathophysiology

Reflux oesophagitis is inflammation of the oesophageal mucosa resulting from exposure to gastric and/or duodenal fluids. The lower oesophagus normally acts as a very effective valve, derangement of which allows acid and pepsin to pass up into the lower oesophagus. Inflamed and damaged oesophageal mucosa is more sensitive than normal to acid so that pain is produced when even dilute acid solutions are perfused over its surface. Furthermore, the damaged oesophagus seems less able to 'clear' acid because motor activity is disturbed, and so a vicious circle may be set up.

If duodenogastric reflux is also present, bile can find its way back into the oesophagus. This is probably even more damaging to the mucosa than acid and pepsin alone.

Hiatus hernia may be associated with gastro-oesophageal reflux, but the two conditions do not necessarily occur together. The presence of a hiatus hernia is probably not of great significance in itself, although the "rolling" (type II, para-oesophageal) type of hernia is said to strangulate not infrequently, and large fixed "sliding" hiatus hernias often contain peptic ulcers which bleed.

The lower oesophageal sphincter (LOS) is a region of increased tone of the circular muscle surrounding the lower few centimetres of the oesophagus. Diminished pressures are detected manometrically in this sphincter in patients suffering from reflux. Sphincter control is complex (see Table 1.1). Many gastrointestinal hormones modulate LOS pressure but no specific abnormality explains why reflux oesophagitis is so common.

Diagnosis

The diagnosis is essentially a clinical one, based on the history. There is no specific diagnostic test.

Table 1.1. Agents which influence lower oesophageal sphincter pressure [Castell DO (1975) Ann Intern Med 83: 390–401]

Agents producing decreased lower oesophageal sphincter pressure	Agents producing increased lower oesophageal sphincter pressure
Secretin	Gastrin/pentagastrin
Cholecystokinin	Prostaglandin $F_{2\alpha}$
Glucagon	α-Adrenergic agonists (noradrenaline, phenylephrine)
Prostaglandins E_1, E_2, A_2	
β-Adrenergic agonists (isoprenaline)	Cholinergic (bethanechol, methacholine)
α-Adrenergic antagonists (phentolamine)	Anticholinesterase (edrophonium)
Anticholinergic (atropine)	Betazole
Theophylline	Gastric alkalinisation
Caffeine	Metoclopramide
Gastric acidification	Protein meal
Fatty meal	
Chocolate	
Smoking	
Ethanol	

Clinical Features

Belching is too common and non-specific a symptom to be helpful diagnostically.

1. Symptoms due to acid reflux. These include posturally related chest pain (worse on bending, stooping or lying flat), heartburn and regurgitation of fluid. Chest pain can closely mimic angina. The symptoms may be rapidly relieved by antacids.
2. Symptoms due to complications
   a) Bleeding—with or without discrete peptic ulceration
   b) Stricture formation
   c) Cephalad displacement of the squamomucosal junction (Barrett's oesophagus)

Thus patients may present with (a) acute upper gastrointestinal haemorrhage, (b) haematemesis and/or melaena or (c) insidious bleeding with iron deficiency anaemia and occult blood in the faeces. Dysphagia may simply be related to oesophagitis, but when there is progressive difficulty in swallowing solid food, especially bread and meat, a stricture should be suspected, and neoplasia must be excluded. Patients may present with purely pulmonary problems—recurrent bouts of bronchitis or pneumonia, or a lung abscess. Oesophageal reflux may trigger attacks of asthma in some susceptible subjects.

Barium Swallow

This will show whether a hiatus hernia is present. Spontaneously occurring gastro-oesophageal reflux observed by an experienced radiologist is a useful finding. However, this only occurs in a minority of patients. This has led to the introduction of various provocation tests—head tilt, pressure on abdomen and swallowing of water in head-down position (water siphon test). These are of limited value, as gastro-oesophageal reflux can be induced in 100% of patients when these techniques are applied with sufficient vigour.

Modern double-contrast techniques will show early changes of oesophagitis, with fine serration of the margin and perturbation of coating. Barium studies remain the most useful initial investigation in oesophageal stricture and they are helpful in planning therapy.

Radio-isotope Studies

Gastro-oesophageal reflux can be demonstrated by scanning over the oesophagus after the patient has swallowed an isotopic marker (usually ^{99}Tc-labelled colloid). This technique is little used but has considerable potential.

pH Probe

Overnight monitoring of the pH within the oesophagus is possibly the most sensitive means of detecting gastro-oesophageal reflux. Some surgeons require this test to be positive before they will undertake anti-reflux surgery.

Reproduction of Symptoms

The above tests may indicate that reflux is taking place, but they do not indicate that symptoms are related to reflux. The *Bernstein test*, in which dilute acid is introduced into the oesophagus, is simple to perform, and occasionally of value in demonstrating to both patient and physician that symptoms are due to contact of sensitive mucosa and acid. It is of particular value when chest pain mimics angina.

Demonstration of Oesophagitis

Oesophagitis may be obvious on inspection endoscopically, with hyperaemia and friability of the mucosa. Endoscopy is the only reliable means of establishing oesophagitis as the cause of gastrointestinal haemorrhage. Strictures can be visualised, brushed and biopsied and dilated, on a single occasion if desired. The Z line is an abrupt demarcation between the pink velvety squamous mucosa of the oesophagus and the red fleshy columnar epithelium of the stomach. This line usually occurs at about 38 cm from the teeth, some 2 cm above the diaphragmatic hiatus. Prolonged reflux may be associated with migration of the squamomucosal junction in a cephalad direction. Islands of columnar epithelium may occur in the lower oesophagus. This finding can be confirmed histologically. In the most extreme cases the whole oesophagus may come to be lined by columnar epithelium (Barrett's oesophagus). This condition is thought to be premalignant.

When the oesophagus appears normal macroscopically, biopsy may still be helpful. Even if classical changes of inflammation are not seen, there may be subtler changes with thickening of the basal layer and elongated dermal pegs extending almost to the free surface.

Treatment

Treatment may be divided into medical and surgical, as follows:
Medical
1. Non-drug methods
   a) Postural measures
   b) Weight reduction
   c) Avoidance of fats
   d) Cessation of smoking
2. Increase in LOS pressure
   a) Metoclopramide (or domperidone)
   b) Bethanechol
3. Modification of reflux fluid
   a) Antacids±alginate
      ±carbenoxolone
   b) H$_2$ receptor blockers

Surgical
1. Reduction of hiatus hernia
2. Anti-reflux measures

Postural Measures

Sufferers from reflux oesophagitis should be advised to adopt postures which retain acid in the stomach by gravity. During the day this involves avoidance of bending and stooping—a physiotherapist may be able to suggest new working methods or long-handled tools or to retrain the patient to bend the knees rather than the back. Similarly patients are advised to avoid tight clothing as external compression of the abdomen will produce gastro-oesophageal reflux. The effectiveness of such measures has been little studied but they are cheap and harmless.

Traditionally patients are also advised to elevate the head of the bed. This seems to permit more rapid clearance of acid from the oesophagus. There is no consensus as to the degree of elevation, suggestions ranging from 4 in. to 28 cm. Many patients complain that this causes them to slip down or fall out of the bottom of the bed. Silk pyjamas may make this worse. The author is not aware of any study of the effect of these practices on marital harmony!

Other Non-drug Remedies

Smoking has been shown to diminish LOS pressure and patients should be advised to desist. Other prohibitions for the same reason include avoidance of fatty food, chocolate and alcohol. Coffee, orange and tomato juice may worsen heartburn by a direct irritant effect on an inflamed oesophageal mucosa. Many patients appear to benefit from weight reduction.

Antacid and Antacid Combinations

If patients' symptoms fail to settle with modifications of life-style, drug therapy may be required. A simple antacid should be tried first. Antacids are effective symptomatic agents. As well as raising the pH of refluxed gastric fluid, they have been shown to raise LOS pressure, possibly by releasing gastrin.

Addition of alginate to antacid (as in Gaviscon or Gastrocote) significantly reduces the number of reflux episodes and the time the oesophagus is exposed to acid. The alginate causes a 'raft' of antacid to float on top of the gastric contents so that if reflux occurs, the fluid brought into contact with the oesophageal mucosa is neutral. Although this concept appears fanciful, there is some evidence that this does in fact occur. A notorious error is to prescribe together an antacid/alginate mixture and a surface tension lowering agent like dimethicone (as in Siloxyl or Polycrol). The surface tension lowering agent will cause the 'raft' to sink. Alginate may also protect the mucosa by plugging the intercellular spaces and preventing the refluxed acid from penetrating the mucosa.

Antacids should not be combined with local anaesthetics as the latter are ineffective in relieving acid induced oesophageal pain. However, antacid can usefully be combined with carbenoxolone (as in Pyrogastrone, which also contains alginate). This is useful in producing symptomatic relief and healing of oesophageal ulcers and inflammation. Unfortunately, although the recommended daily dose of carbenoxolone in this treatment regime is low at 100 mg daily, side-effects of fluid retention and hypokalaemia do occur.

Metoclopramide

Metoclopramide increases LOS pressure when given both intravenously and orally. In addition, oral metoclopramide is effective in reducing heartburn in patients with reflux symptoms. Interestingly, these two effects are poorly corelated.

The long-term use of metoclopramide is complicated by a high incidence of side-effects, especially related to the central nervous system—extrapyramidal manifestations, hyperprolactinaemia, anxiety, nervousness, lassitude and drowsiness being common.

Domperidone

Domperidone is a dopamine antagonist, like metoclopramide. Both drugs increase LOS pressure and accelerate gastric emptying. Early clinical results with domperidone indicate a useful symptomatic effect in patients with reflux oesophagitis. A possible advantage of domperidone is that the drug does not penetrate the blood-brain barrier. It therefore seems relatively free of the CNS side-effects which inhibit long-term use of metoclopramide. Only occasional headaches and urticaria have been noted as significant side-effects. The drug, like all dopamine antagonists, does cause a rise in serum prolactin.

Cimetidine

Cimetidine has been tested in a number of well-controlled clinical trials. The drug is clearly effective in improving symptoms, and probably effective in improving the endoscopic appearance and histological severity of the oesophagitis. It does not reduce the requirement for periodic dilations once an oesophageal stricture is established.

Cimetidine is a drug about which there are reservations with respect to long-term use. This subject is discussed further under maintenance therapy for duodenal ulceration.

Bethanechol

Bethanechol is a cholinergic drug which has been used more in the U.S.A. than in the U.K. It is effective in raising LOS pressure, reducing symptoms and healing oesophagitis. The drug may also produce a more effective peristaltic action in the oesophagus.

Side-effects are predictable—nausea and vomiting, sweating, salivation, lacrimation, frequency of micturition and defaecation, palpitations and flushing. The most troublesome effect clinically is diarrhoea.

Treatment of Complications

Bleeding Oesophagitis and Oesophageal Ulcer

These account for between 3% and 10% of cases of acute upper gastrointestinal haemorrhage. Diffuse oesophageal bleeding is rarely life threatening and will usually stop spontaneously with transfusion and simple supportive measures. Cimetidine is often used, but there is no evidence that it is effective. Somatostatin may be more useful when it becomes generally available.

Oesophageal ulcers occasionally give rise to massive haemorrhage. Trans-catheter arterial embolisation may be effective in causing haemorrhage to cease. Although oesophageal bleeding sites can be cauterised by means of diathermy probes passed down the biopsy channel of an endoscope, this approach cannot be recommended at present, as the risk of perforation of the oesophagus must be high.

Stricture Formation

The management of oesophageal strictures has been revolutionised by techniques employing the flexible fibre-optic endoscope.

Minor strictures may be traversed under direct vision by means of a paediatric-sized endoscope. If this is not possible, a soft-ended guide wire can be passed through the upper end of the stricture. Successful passage of the stricture (so that the flexible tip of the wire enters freely into the stomach) can be checked by fluoroscopy. A preliminary barium swallow should be performed to show the length of the stricture and any associated hiatus hernia. Difficulties may be encountered when the stricture is

1. Long
2. Irregular
3. Sinuous
4. Associated with oesophageal ulceration
5. Associated with a hiatus hernia

When the guide wire is in position it can be used to "railroad" various bougies. The Eder Peustow technique of passing olives of increasing size is highly successful, but can be uncomfortable for the patient. Eder Peustow dilations may be best performed under general anaesthesia, at least on the first occasion. Otherwise, sedation will suffice. The Celestin technique of passing soft tapered bougies is very quick, easy and better tolerated. However, with very long strictures (especially caustic strictures), the Eder Peustow technique is preferable.

The natural history of oesophageal strictures is unpredictable. Most remit after one to three dilations and patients may remain able to swallow comfortably thereafter or require only occasional dilatations. Other strictures obstinately recur. Very rapid and repeated relapse after dilation is characteristic of a malignant stricture and repeated cytological and histological examinations are required. A co-existent oesophageal ulcer seems to make sustained successful dilatation of a stricture less likely.

No drug has been shown to diminish the frequency of requirement for dilations, although it would seem reasonable to treat associated gastro-oesophageal reflux vigorously.

Barrett's Epithelium

Replacement of the normal squamous epithelium lining of the oesophagus by columnar epithelium occurs in patients experiencing severe and continuous reflux. Progressive displacement cephalad of the squamomucosal junction has been observed in the presence of severe reflux, occurring spontaneously and also following surgical resection of the LOS.

The lesion may predispose to adenocarcinoma of the oesophagus. This can be diagnosed at a pre-invasive stage by cytological examination of brushings obtained endoscopically. It is sensible to review annually all patients with Barrett's oesophagus by endoscopy with random biopsies and cytology.

Peptic ulcers occurring within Barrett's epithelium often bleed repeatedly. This may require surgery but cimetidine seems to be effective in preventing bleeding. Intensive antacid therapy appears less effective.

Aspiration

Attacks of asthma may be triggered reflexly when acid enters the lower oesophagus. Considerable relief may follow treatment with cimetidine. H^2 blockers seem to have little effect on airways resistance in normal people, despite evidence for pulmonary H_2 receptors.

Barium may occasionally reflux into the lungs during a barium swallow. Otherwise, recurrent aspiration is a clinical diagnosis and tends to be an indication for surgery. However, if severe pulmonary damage has already been sustained, patients may be a poor operative risk.

Surgery

A discussion of the surgical treatment of reflux oesophagitis is beyond the scope of the present chapter. Indications for operation include complications (intractable bleeding, stricture formation or aspiration) and failure of medical treatment to control severe symptoms. The latter category gives rise to most problems. A range of operative procedures (employing both abdominal and thoracic approaches) are effective in relieving symptoms and increasing LOS pressure. These two effects are not always related. However, there is a significant peri-operative mortality. Postoperative complications include distressing bloating associated with inability to belch or vomit, and there is a tendency for symptoms to relapse after 5–6 years.

Summary

A phased approach to the treatment of reflux oesophagitis has been proposed. A modified scheme is shown below:

Phase I

Modified diet
   Weight reduction if necessary
   Decreased fat, chocolate, alcohol
   Avoid specific precipitating foods
Elevate head of bed
Decrease smoking
Antacids or antacid/alginate mixtures

Phase II

Agents which heal oesophagitis
   Antacid/carbenoxolone mixtures
Agents which decrease gastric acid
   Cimetidine
Agents which raise LOS pressure
   Metoclopramide or domperidone
   Bethanechol

Phase III
Consider surgery

All the drugs listed under phase II have significant side-effects and none could be unreservedly proposed for long-term maintenance therapy. Fortunately, most patients' symptoms settle with minor therapy as outlined in phase I. Even when symptoms are severe, they are frequently intermittent, so that short courses of phase II drugs are appropriate. Only a small minority of patients with unremitting and intractable symptoms or complications need progress to phase III.

Carcinoma of the Oesophagus

Pathophysiology

Very rarely, oesophageal cancer can be inherited in a simple Mendelian dominant manner in association with tylosis (hyperkeratosis palmaris et plantaris). This has been best described in two families in Liverpool, but other pedigrees are on record. Sufferers have a 95% risk of developing the cancer by the age of 65 years.

Patients with coeliac disease have an increased risk of developing lymphoma, and also carcinomata of the gastrointestinal tract, particularly of the oesophagus.

With these exceptions there is a striking lack of evidence of any genetic predisposition to the disease. Carcinoma of the oesophagus is no commoner amongst first-degree relatives of a victim than amongst the general population. This and the geographical distribution of the disease strongly suggest an environmental factor. Very high incidences are found in Iran and China, and an "epidemic" of the condition has occurred over the last half-century in South Africa.

Associations with the disorder include a higher incidence amongst smokers and those who drink alcohol. Lye strictures are notorious for late development of carcinoma. Achalasia of the cardia also appears to be premalignant. Interestingly, the carcinomas which develop are frequently in the mid-oesphagus, and may occur even long after surgical relief of the obstruction.

Adenocarcinoma

Most so-called adenocarcinomas of the oesophagus are growths which arise from the cardia of the stomach and invade the lower oesophagus. These tumours are normally dealt with surgically, although inoperable lesions can be intubated endoscopically. True adenocarcinoma of the oesophagus is rare, probably representing 1% of all cancers of the organ. This lesion arises in islands of columnar epithelium or in Barrett's oesophagus, both of which are associated with reflux oesophagitis.

All tumours of the oesophagus should be biopsied and classified as adenocarcinoma, squamous carcinoma or undifferentiated. The latter two are radiosensitive. Adenocarcinoma should be surgically resected.

Postcricoid Carcinoma

This is commoner in females and may be related to iron deficiency anaemia (Plummer-Vinson or Paterson-Brown-Kelly syndrome), although this association is becoming rare. Carcinoma in this site affects a rather younger age group than more distal lesions. There is little doubt that this group is best treated by radiotherapy.

Squamous Carcinoma of the Thoracic Oesophagus

Although the mean interval between onset of symptoms and diagnosis is surprisingly long (7.5 months in Britain), there is no evidence that survival is related to length of history. The operative mortality is 29%. Of all the factors studied, the most useful prognostically is the length of the stricture. Lesions longer than 8 cm are almost certainly unresectable, and those longer than 6 cm are generally incurable.

There has never been a controlled trial of radiotherapy versus surgery for this disease. Radiotherapy is generally reserved for those patients with extensive disease or those who are unfit for surgery. In spite of this, the 1-year survival rate following radiotherapy is 18%. This is not dissimilar to that of surgically treated patients and it avoids the operative mortality. The 5-year survival rate for radiotherapy is 6%, which compares favourably with 4% using surgical management.

Apart from crude survival statistics, we have few measures of efficacy of any treatment offered. Hardly any patients return to work after a resection. After surgery, 30% may experience recurrent dysphagia and 20% need dilatations. This is both because of unresected carcinoma at the margins of the anastomosis and because of fibrous stricturing. With radiotherapy, dysphagia may get worse during or immediately after treatment. It is impossible to anticipate which patients will experience this. Up to 50% will require oesophageal dilations. Endoscopic intubation is not recommended prior to radiotherapy, but a fine-bore feeding tube may be positioned in case obstruction occurs. Endoscopic dilatation and tube emplacement may be helpful if post-radiation stricturing occurs.

At present it is impossible to lay down dogmatic guidelines for therapy, but the broad position can be summarised:

1. All patients should undergo investigations for distant metastases, including liver scan, bronchoscopy and CT scan where practicable. The patient with secondaries is doomed and should be treated palliatively with endoscopic dilatations and emplacement of a Celestin-type tube. This carries a mortality of about 12.5% (roughly equally due to perforation and aspiration pneumonia), but if successful gives excellent palliation.

2. The fit patient with a distal lesion less than 5 cm in length has the best chance of surviving operation, and this should probably be offered. Pre-operative nutritional support may be helpful.

3. Other patients should be considered for megavoltage radiotherapy, usually in the form of 5000 rad given over 4 weeks in 20 days of treatment at 250 rad each day.

4. The role of chemotherapy (usually bleomycin or cis-platin) is undefined.

Oesophageal Varices

Pathophysiology

Oesophageal variceal haemorrhage is associated with a hospital admission mortality of up to 60% (as compared with an overall death rate from acute upper gastrointestinal haemorrhage of 8%–10%). Varices result from enlargement of collateral vessels shunting blood from the portal circulation to the systemic venous system in portal hypertension. These enlarged venous networks lie particularly superficially in the lower oesophagus, over a region extending a few centimetres above the squamomucosal junction. It is at this site that haemorrhage is especially prone to occur.

The cardinal physical sign of portal hypertension is splenomegaly.

In the U.K., portal hypertension is usually secondary to liver disease, commonly cirrhosis. In a minority of cases portal hypertension results from extrahepatic causes (usually portal vein thrombosis) or non- or precirrhotic liver disease. Prognosis and management are dictated by the functional state of the liver, so this should be initially assessed at the bedside.

Varices are commonly present in portal hypertension, but they do not necessarily bleed. It is not possible to predict accurately which varices will bleed, but there is a greater risk of bleeding if the varices are large. There is no simple relationship between the pressure in the portal system and the risk of bleeding.

It has been suggested that varices bleed because the thin-walled vessels rupture under high pressure. Alternatively, an episode of bleeding might be precipitated by peptic erosion of the mucosa overlying a varix. There is little to support the latter theory, and cimetidine is ineffective in preventing variceal haemorrhage.

Treatment Strategy

Since bleeding is unpredictable, and may not occur, the mere discovery of varices does not, in itself, necessitate treatment. However, having bled once, recurrent haemorrhage is very likely. Treatment is therefore appropriate in two situations:

1. Control of acute bleeding
2. Prevention of rebleeding

Acute Bleeding

Diagnosis

All patients with suspected variceal haemorrhage should undergo endoscopy to confirm the source of bleeding as soon as they have been adequately resuscitated. Cirrhotics, particularly alcoholics, may be bleeding from acute gastric erosions, Mallory-Weiss tears or peptic ulcers, as well as from their varices. Occasionally an actively bleeding point may be visualised. If a fresh clot is visible on a varix which is not easily washed off, a presumptive diagnosis of variceal bleeding can be made, especially if no other likely bleeding source is seen in the upper gastrointestinal tract.

Cirrhotic patients may have clotting defects, so that the prothrombin time should be urgently determined. It is wise to give vitamin K 10 mg parenterally in all bleeding patients with known or suspected liver disease, and to repeat this if the prothrombin time is prolonged. Similarly, patients with portal hypertension may have hypersplenism with thrombocytopenia, so that a platelet count should be urgently performed.

General Management

Ruptured oesophageal varices often lead to massive bleeding, and urgent restoration of circulating blood volume is the first essential. An intravenous infusion should be set up immediately. If the patient has known or suspected liver disease, saline infusions should be avoided, as such patients may retain sodium and water, and peripheral oedema and/or ascites will be worsened. In this circumstance 5% dextrose can be infused initially. Plasma expanders such as Haemaccel can be used whilst blood is being urgently cross-matched, but they contain large amounts of sodium. Similarly, fresh-frozen plasma can be given, and this is particularly useful in patients with liver disease with clotting defects.

Blood transfusion requirements are frequently massive in variceal haemorrhage. Precautions must therefore be taken to avoid the deleterious consequences: Blood should be as fresh as possible, warmed and filtered and an injection of 10 ml calcium gluconate given intravenously with every two units of transfused blood. Transfusion requirements are frequently underestimated clinically, and it is wise to monitor the central venous pressure.

In all patients with liver disease (usually cirrhosis) who are bleeding from oesophageal varices, the prognosis depends on the degree of liver cell failure. A formal assessment of this can be made using the Child's grading (see Table 1.2).

Table 1.2. Child's grading of liver function

	A	B	C
Serum bilirubin (μmol/dl)	<35	35–50	>50
Serum albumin (g/l)	>35	30–35	<30
Ascites	None	Easily controlled	Poorly controlled
Neurological disorder	None	Minimal	Coma
Nutrition	Excellent	Good	Wasting

A severe gastrointestinal bleed in a patient with established liver disease is a potent stimulus to the development of hepatic pre-coma or coma. All patients at risk should be put on to a hepatic failure regime, as outlined in Chap. 8. Many more patients die of irreversible liver failure than from uncontrolled or unceasing haemorrhage.

Measures to Arrest Variceal Bleeding

Drugs

General measures to resuscitate the patient, to restore circulating blood volume, and to contain liver cell failure are probably more important than specific measures to stop bleeding. Many haemorrhages will stop spontaneously. When faced with continued bleeding, the simplest means of control is with a Pitressin infusion. A single injection of 20 units of Pitressin, freshly made up in 100 ml 5% dextrose, can be given over 10 min. This is contra-indicated in severe ischaemic heart disease. Administration of the drug causes pallor, abdominal colic and defaecation (usually fresh melaena), especially if the agent is infused too rapidly. It is preferable to set up a constant infusion of vasopressin into a peripheral vein, increasing the rate slowly from 0.1 unit/minute to a maximum of 1.0 unit/minute until haemorrhage is controlled. There appears to be no clinical benefit in increasing the infusion rate above this range, and if 30 min at 1.0 unit/minute fails to control bleeding, the method should be abandoned. Intra-arterial administration conveys no benefit over intravenous usage.

Vasopressin may shortly be superceded by Gly-pressin, which has a longer half-life and is consequently much easier to administer. Somatostatin may have a role in this situation, but this drug has not been adequately investigated and is not generally available.

Physical Methods

Balloon tamponade is a hazardous but potentially life-saving procedure. Meticulous attention to technique is essential. Most U.K. centres utilise the Minnesota 4 lumen tube or a Sengstaken-Blakemore tube, modified by taping a nasogastric tube to the device so that secretions can be continuously aspirated above the oesophageal balloon. Without this modification, aspiration pneumonia is inevitable.

Modern latex tubes are very floppy even when kept in a refrigerator. Accordingly the author prefers to "tow" the tube into position using an endoscope. A pair of forceps is passed through the biopsy channel of the instrument. The distal end of the tube is then seized in the jaws of the forceps (the side holes for gastric aspiration are convenient for this), after which the tube is introduced alongside the endoscope, and the whole assembly passed into the stomach. The jaws are released and the forceps withdrawn. The stomach balloon is partially or completely inflated before the endoscope is withdrawn. This prevents the Sengstaken-Blakemore tube coming up with the endoscope. Furthermore, the correct position of the inflated gastric balloon filling the gastric fundus can be checked visually.

It is a common mistake to underestimate the capacity of the gastric balloon. It should be inflated to 200–250 ml. Many authorities use air, but distending the balloon with liquid has the advantage that the same volume can be accurately withdrawn. This precludes the risk of an incompletely deflated balloon being pulled up through the cardia, oesophagus and pharynx. A convenient liquid is water-soluble contrast medium diluted with water or saline. This permits the position of the gastric balloon to be checked radiologically. When the balloon is inflated, the tube is drawn up so that the veins feeding the oesophageal varices are compressed in the gastric fundus. The oesophageal balloon is then inflated with air to a pressure of 45–60 mmHg. This pressure must be continuously monitored. The pharynx and upper oesophagus must be continuously aspirated when the balloons are in place. The gastric tube can be aspirated continuously or discontinuously. The upper end of the tube is brought out through the mouth and taped to the cheek. Traction should not be used.

A Sengstaken-Blakemore tube is very uncomfortable, both during introduction and whilst in position. However, many patients with liver disease will be obtunded or comatose during a severe variceal bleed. Patients who are alert find the tube an ordeal, but sedation or analgesics should be avoided if at all possible. These agents will have a prolonged time course and may provoke hepatic encephalopathy.

The oesophageal balloon must be deflated within 36 h, and preferably 24 h, to prevent damage to the oesophagus, possibly with ulceration. Many patients rebleed when the cuff is deflated. Consequently, it is important to plan the next therapeutic manoeuvre carefully.

Sclerotherapy

Sclerotherapy was originally pioneered using the rigid oesophagoscope, but has now become more widely practised using the flexible fibre-optic endoscopy. The technique is effective both in stopping active bleeding and in preventing rebleeding.

Various sclerosing fluids have been used, including ethanolamine oleate, phenol, sodium morrhuate and sodium tetradecyl sulphate (at concentrations of both 3% and 1%). A wide range of dosage has been used—from 0.5 to 5 ml of the various fluids at each of several injection sites. Injections have been made in a variety of sites, from a ring just above the squamomucosal junction to throughout the oesophagus. Injections into the varices, submucosally alongside the varices and submucosally away from the varices have all been advocated.

Despite the variety of techniques described, sclerotherapy has been enthusiastically taken up and has replaced surgical portosystemic shunting as the procedure of choice for prevention of rebleeding.

Injection of varices may not be feasible, however, in the presence of severe active bleeding, or may fail to arrest the haemorrhage. Embolisation or transection procedures should then be considered.

Embolisation

The portal venous system can be entered by the percutaneous transhepatic route, using a cholangiography needle. By this means, a catheter-over-guide wire assembly can be advanced, under fluoroscopic control, to the veins supplying oesophageal varices (left gastric and short gastric vessels). These vessels can be obliterated by injecting suitable material (Gelfoam or minute wire coils).

This technique has been successful in arresting acute variceal haemorrhage, but there is a high rate of recurrent bleeding over the following weeks. Therefore one should undertake some other procedure to prevent rebleeding, e.g. sclerotherapy, β-blockade, devascularisation procedures or shunting.

Embolisation requires a high degree of technical expertise which is not generally available.

Devascularisation Procedures

Operative transection of the oesophagus has been greatly simplified by the introduction of the stapling gun. At operation the abdomen is opened, the lower oesophagus mobilised, and the vagi dissected free. The stapling gun is introduced into the stomach, via a gastrotomy, and directed into the lower oesophagus. A ligature is tied around the lower oesophagus, drawing a ring of tissue into the jaws of the device. Then the gun is fired. This causes instantaneous resection of a cylinder of lower oesophagus, and anastomosis of the cut ends by a ring of staples. This obliterates all venous channels at the lower oesophageal level.

This procedure is fast, easy and relatively safe. Some authorities combine it with a more extensive surgical devascularisation around the cardia. It is probably the procedure of choice in variceal haemorrhage uncontrolled by non-operative means. There is, however, a significant risk of the development of recurrent varices and eventual rebleeding.

Emergency Shunt Procedures

Emergency portocaval shunting to control acute exsanguinating haemorrhage is associated with unacceptable mortality. There may be a role for shunt operations in patients who continue to bleed or who bleed repeatedly despite the use of lesser measures. In this setting, many authorities would favour a simple operative procedure such as an interposition 'H' graft of Dacron. However, many such shunts fail to remain patent.

Prevention of Rebleeding

After variceal haemorrhage has stopped either spontaneously or following the procedures outlined above, consideration should be given to preventing further episodes of bleeding. In this context, therapeutic possibilities include:

1. Injection sclerotherapy
2. β-blockade
3. Shunt procedures

Injection Sclerotherapy

Patients may be given a course of injections to obliterate their oesophageal varices. This usually requires about six injections. The first two or three can be performed during the initial hospital admission at intervals of a few days. Thereafter the injections can be repeated at approximately monthly intervals until the varicosities are no longer visible at oesophagoscopy. Follow-up endoscopies are then performed at 6–12 month intervals, and any recurrent varices injected. Rigid oesophagoscopy requires general anaesthesia, and general anaesthesia may be preferable if an overtube is used, but many centres prefer to use flexible endoscopic techniques under diazepam sedation. Complications include those of the anaesthetic and/or endoscopy itself (perforation, inhalation), and also strictures, ulceration (if large volumes are injected submucosally), retrosternal pain and pleural effusions.

β-Blockade

β-Blockers, especially propranolol, will lower portal pressure and have been shown to reduce the incidence of rebleeding from oesophageal varices. Propranolol is given in a dose from 40 mg to 360 mg twice daily by mouth in order to reduce resting heart rate by 25%. The method is still under investigation, but may prove the simplest means of dealing with this situation.

Operative Shunt Procedures

These formed the standard treatment until recent years. The conventional end-to-side portacaval shunt is fairly simple to perform, but in contrast to injection sclerotherapy does not prolong survival. A successful shunt protects from bleeding, but liver function deteriorates and patients frequently succumb from hepatic failure. There is also a high risk of chronic portosystemic encephalopathy, even in the presence of good liver function.

The distal splenorenal or Warren shunt may be associated with a reduced risk of portosystemic encephalopathy, but is technically difficult, not universally applicable and remains controversial.

Further Reading

Clark AW, MacDougall BRD, Westaby D, Mitchell KJ, Silk DBA, Strunin L, Dawson JL, Williams R (1980) Prospective controlled trial of injection sclerotherapy in patients with cirrhosis and recent variceal haemorrhage. Lancet II: 552–554

Fox S, Beher J (1979) Control of lower oesophageal sphincter pressure and acid reflux. Clin Gastroenterol 8(1): 37–52

Lebrac D, Poynard T, Millar P, Benhamon JP (1981) Propranolol for prevention of recurrent gastrointestinal bleeding in patients with cirrhosis. N Engl J Med 305: 1371–1374

2 Peptic Ulcer Disease

R. A. Mountford

Duodenal Ulceration

Pathophysiology

Genetic Factors

Duodenal ulceration occurs more frequently in patients of blood group O who are non-secretors. This association seems to concern duodenal ulcers which become manifest in middle age or later. Late onset duodenal ulcers are more virulent, with increased risk of complications. On the other hand, patients with duodenal ulceration presenting in the first two decades of life are more likely to be of blood groups A, B or AB and to have a strong family history of peptic ulceration.

There is an association between HLA B5 status and duodenal ulceration, at least in white males.

Elevated serum group 1 pepsinogen may be a marker for some types of duodenal ulceration.

Prevalence

Duodenal ulcer remains predominantly a disease of males, but the difference in incidence between the sexes has fallen since earlier this century. The prevalence is highest (approximately 10%) for males aged 45–54. However, the disease is probably becoming less common overall, having "peaked" in the early 1950s.

Duodenal ulceration is more common in the elderly than is generally realised: 20% of endoscopically proven duodenal ulcers occur in patients over 65 years old.

There is undoubtedly a higher incidence amongst cigarette smokers.

The disease is roughly equally represented in all socio-economic groups.

Associated Diseases

There is an association between duodenal ulceration and the following diseases:

1. Chronic renal failure (especially in patients undergoing haemodialysis or following renal transplantation)
2. Hyperparathyroidism
3. Cirrhosis
4. Cardiovascular disease (especially arteriosclerotic coronary heart disease and aortic valve disease)
5. Chronic respiratory disease

Natural History

The mortality due to duodenal ulcer has been falling for 40 years. Several studies suggest that duodenal ulceration tends to be a self-limiting disease with severe symptoms occurring typically over a period of 10–15 years, following which spontaneous remission occurs.

It has been estimated that 7% of patients with duodenal ulcer will die of their disease. Over one-half of these deaths are due to complications (especially haemorrhage); the remainder are post-operative.

Diagnosis

Clinical Features

The symptomatology of duodenal ulceration has been investigated as part of a computer study of patients with "dyspepsia". One striking finding was that the pain of duodenal ulceration appears unrelated to meals in the majority of patients.

Investigations

Double-contrast barium radiology can achieve comparable accuracy to endoscopy in diagnosing duodenal ulceration. However, it remains difficult in some instances for the radiologist to demonstrate an ulcer crater, especially when the duodenal cap is already deformed by previous scarring. This is important since endoscopic follow-up studies have shown that up to 50% of ulcer relapses are asymptomatic, at least initially. The clinical significance of an asymptomatic relapse is uncertain, but in 10% of gastrointestinal bleeds attributed to peptic ulceration, the ulcer may be painless. Similarly, up to 17% of perforations occur in patients with no significant dyspepsia previously. It could therefore be argued that the patient is only safe from these complications if he has no ulcer crater. As one cannot rely upon symptoms, it is logical that the duodenum should be regularly inspected. This is most reliably done by endoscopy.

These issues have become more pertinent since the advent of very effective drugs to heal duodenal ulcers. What is lacking is any consensus regarding prevention of relapse.

Treatment

General (Non-drug) Measures

Diet

No specific diet has a role in improving symptoms or in accelerating healing of a peptic ulcer. Many patients note that their symptoms are worsened by fatty or spicy food and it is common sense for such foods to be avoided. There is no evidence that milk is particularly beneficial in controlling symptoms or in raising intragastric pH.

Cigarette Smoking

Duodenal ulcers are commoner in cigarette smokers, and heal more slowly if patients continue to smoke. This is true regardless of whether patients are treated with an active ulcer healing drug or with a placebo. Patients should be urged strongly to give up the habit.

Alcohol

Patients frequently ask whether they should drink. Concentrated alcohol can cause damage to and bleeding of the gastric mucosa. It is sensible, therefore, to curtail the drinking of spirits, but to make no other prohibition.

Bed Rest

In contrast to gastric ulcer, bed rest does not hasten healing of duodenal ulcers. With modern therapy, treatment of uncomplicated duodenal ulceration is almost exclusively ambulatory.

Symptomatic Drug Treatment

Antacids

Small doses of antacids are traditionally used for symptomatic relief. Curiously, when submitted to double-blind trials, antacids have little if any advantage over placebo in relieving symptoms. However, the huge quantities of proprietary antacids which are sold attest the enduring popularity of this group of drugs. Used intermittently and in small doses the non-absorbed antacids are safe. Patients are undoubtedly grateful to be supplied with antacids to use when their symptoms are severe.

Used in this way, the neutralising capacity of the medicament and the optimal form and timing of dosage to raise intragastric pH are largely irrelevant. The overriding considerations are patient acceptability and convenience. Tablets are certainly more convenient to carry than liquids. There is a wide range to choose from. Patient preference has been little studied, but Maalox was favoured in one study.

Anticholinergics

Anticholinergic drugs, traditionally atropine and propantheline, have been used in duodenal ulceration on the basis that they inhibit basal and stimulated gastric acid secretion and reduce gastric motility. The disadvantage of these agents is that at dosages effective in lowering gastric acid secretion, marked side-effects occur. These are predictable anticholinergic effects of dry mouth, blurred vision, photophobia, constipation, tachycardia, difficulty with micturition and occasionally impotence. This class of drug is contra-indicated in glaucoma, prostatic enlargement and pyloric stenosis, and anticholinergics need to be used with care in cardiac disease where tachycardia might be dangerous.

Anticholinergics have now been superceded, and are rarely used. However, prescribing fashions change in the light of new evidence. Two quaternary ammonium drugs—anisotropine methylbromide and prifinium bromide—are claimed to accelerate ulcer healing and merit further investigation. Unfortunately, the high incidence of side-effects, like dry mouth, makes a truly double-blind trial almost impossible with this class of drugs.

Drugs to Promote Ulcer Healing

Cimetidine

There is no doubt that H_2 receptor blockers have revolutionised the acute healing of duodenal ulcers. In very large numbers of endoscopically monitored, double-blind controlled trials a course of cimetidine (0.8–2.0 g/day) over 4–6 weeks results in 70%–85% healing compared with 30%–40% in the placebo group. This now provides a standard against which other agents must be tested.

Symptomatic improvement is rapid and in many cases dramatic. Antacid requirements are reduced.

The drug appears to be safe. It has been given in enormous overdosage—12 g per day for 5 days—with no ill-effects. Indeed, the patient's duodenal ulcer healed and remained so for at least 4 months. Gynaecomastia occurs uncommonly. Intravenous injection of cimetidine invariably produces rises in serum prolactin concentrations. This effect is probably related to transiently high serum levels of cimetidine, as it is not always observed following oral administration of the drug. Similarly, elevated serum levels of prolactin,

FSH, LH and oestradiol have been observed in some male patients complaining of impotence whilst taking the drug. Gonadal atrophy is observed in male rats exposed to large doses of the drug over prolonged periods. Some of these effects may be due to competitive binding of the drug to androgen receptor sites. Gynaecomastia usually regresses on withdrawal of the drug. The anti-androgen effect appears to be specific to cimetidine rather than a characteristic of H_2 blockers as a group.

Mental clouding can occur with confusion, delirium, psychosis, hypomania, hallucinations and agitation. These effects appear limited to elderly patients who are severely ill, especially those in chronic renal failure.

Some patients show transient rises of serum creatinine and uric acid on commencing therapy. Rare instances of interstitial nephritis have been reported. Cimetidine potentiates warfarin, phenytoin and the benzodiazepines. Occasionally patients need to be withdrawn from the drug because of rashes, diarrhoea, headache, nausea and vomiting, myalgia or dizziness.

Overall, the toxic effects are trivial when compared with the huge amounts of the drug currently being prescribed. More importantly, the bone marrow depression which rendered unusable the parent drug, metiamide, occurs rarely if ever with cimetidine.

Anxiety and controversy over cimetidine therapy centre on the risk of carcinogenicity. Under normal conditions (i.e. acid pH) the stomach is essentially sterile. However, if the stomach is rendered achlorhydric, it can become colonised by bacteria. This has been shown to occur with cimetidine therapy. Bacteria can convert dietary nitrate via nitrite to N-nitroso compounds. These are strongly carcinogenic in animals. This is one theory to explain the increased incidence of gastric carcinoma in various clinical states in which gastric acid secretion is impaired, i.e. pernicious anaemia and following partial gastrectomy.

The alleged risks with cimetidine are twofold.

1. The drug renders the stomach relatively alkaline for long periods.
2. The drug itself can be readily nitrosylated to N-nitrosocimetidine.

Concern has become heightened recently by the finding of elevated N-nitrosamine concentrations in gastric juice following the administration of cimetidine. This requires confirmation, especially as no methodology for assaying N-nitroso compounds is universally accepted.

Cimetidine in conventional doses reduces gastric acidity, but by no means produces achlorhydria throughout the 24 hours. Gastric acid recovers, particularly preprandially and during the night. Nitrosylation is of uncertain significance as the same phenomenon occurs with many other commonly used medicaments. Although cases of gastric carcinoma have been reported in patients taking cimetidine, no definite causal relationship has emerged. Extensive animal testing has failed to demonstrate carcinogenesis despite prolonged exposure to high doses of the drug.

At present there is no evidence to suggest that short courses of cimetidine carry any enhanced risk of carcinoma. Many clinicians, however, have reservations about using the drug long-term for prophylaxis. This problem is discussed further under "Maintenance Therapy".

Other H_2 Receptor Blockers

Ranitidine is a newer H_2 blocker which differs from others in the group by having a furan, rather than an imidazole or thiazole, ring structure. It is four to five times more potent than cimetidine on a molar basis. Studies have shown ranitidine 100 mg or 150 mg twice daily to be equally as effective in healing duodenal ulcers as cimetidine 200 mg three times a day and 400 mg at night. Oxmetidine is another long-acting H_2 blocker with the advantage of twice-daily dosage; however, it is not yet available.

In fact, cimetidine can be given as 400 mg twice daily rather than as 1 g spaced through the day. There is no significant difference in effectiveness between the two regimes on testing. Thus 400 mg twice daily can be recommended as being cheaper, and one would anticipate better patient compliance.

Colloidal Bismuth

Colloidal bismuth (usually tripotassium dicitrato bismuthate—De-Nol) has a complex mode of action within the stomach. It has an antacid effect, inactivates pepsin and may stimulate secretion of mucus. Probably its most important effect, however, is the precipitation of bismuth oxide at acid pH. This substance forms a tenacious protective layer on mucosal surface, which is resistant to pepsin and acid. Bismuth oxide has a particular affinity for granulation tissue, as in an ulcer base. It has been observed to stay within an ulcer crater for several days and is thought to permit the underlying processes of ulcer healing to take place.

Because precipitation only takes place at acid pH, De-Nol is best taken on an empty stomach, and milk, food and antacids should be avoided for about an hour. For this reason, simultaneous therapy with De-Nol and cimetidine appears irrational.

De-Nol's effectiveness in healing duodenal ulcers is supported by several well-controlled studies.

One disadvantage of the liquid preparation is its abominable taste. A much more palatable tablet preparation which appears as effective as the liquid form is now available. Both forms of the drug may stain the mouth and turn the stools dark in colour, mimicking melaena. Sucralfate (antepsin) is an aluminium based compound which seems to work rather similarly to colloidal bismuth. It may prove to have greater patient acceptability.

Cases of neurotoxicity have been described following ingestion of bismuth subgallate, which was previously used to reduce volumes of colostomy or ileostomy effluent. However, there is some dispute as to whether this toxicity was related to the bismuth or to the subgallate moeity. Furthermore, absorption of bismuth from De-Nol is small, although measurable. The anion is promptly excreted in the urine without a significant rise in blood level.

Of particular interest is the claim that the relapse rate of ulcers healed by De-Nol is markedly less than that of those treated with cimetidine. In one study, 23 of 27 patients had relapsed 12 months following cimetidine therapy whereas this occurred in only 11 of 30 De-Nol treated patients.

This apparent protective effect of De-Nol may be related to the return of ultrastructural normality of the duodenal mucosal cells which occurs following 6 weeks' therapy. By contrast, the mucosa remains abnormal after treatment with cimetidine, even after a year at a dosage of 400 mg twice daily. De-Nol appears to promote growth of microvilli, diminution of inflammatory changes and increase in numbers of goblet cells with secretion of a protective mucin layer.

Carbenoxolone

Initially the efficacy of carbenoxolone in the treatment of duodenal ulceration was doubted, but recent trials have demonstrated convincingly that the drug is effective. Nevertheless, it cannot be recommended as first-line therapy because of the high incidence of side-effects, especially salt and water retention, with oedema, hypertension and heart failure, and hypokalaemia. These effects appear commoner and are more troublesome in the older age group, and in practice the drug cannot be recommended in patients over 60 years of age.

No information is available on interaction between carbenoxolone and diuretics in the healing of duodenal ulcers (cf. gastric ulcer). All patients commencing carbenoxolone therapy need careful monitoring. They should be seen at least every 2 weeks, examined for signs of fluid retention, have their weight and blood pressure checked and have their serum potassium level measured.

There has been a suggestion that carbenoxolone-healed ulcers relapse less rapidly than cimetidine-healed ulcers. Carbenoxolone has also been used successfully to maintain healing in ulcers treated with cimetidine as well as in ulcers healed by carbenoxolone itself.

Intensive Antacid Regimes

The alleged symptomatic benefit of small doses of antacids has been mentioned. In large doses, however, antacids accelerate healing of duodenal ulcers. In order to achieve this, very large quantities of powerful antacids have to be given. Liquids neutralise more acid than tablets in conventional dosage. Typically 30 ml of an antacid mixture is given seven times a day: 1 h and 3 h after each meal and once at night.

A wide range of commercial antacids are available. Some are combined with surface tension-lowering agents like dimethicone, or with alginates or peppermint oil. They vary widely in their neutralising capacity.

Magnesium—aluminium mixtures are probably the best choice. Soluble antacids like sodium bicarbonate cause problems of alkalosis and the effects of a large sodium load. Calcium carbonate produces rebound hyperacidity and may cause hypercalcaemia and impaired renal function.

Aluminium hydroxide may produce constipation, phosphate depletion (anorexia, weakness, bone pain) and possibly progressive neurological impairment in patients with renal failure. Magnesium hydroxide or trisilicate may produce diarrhoea and also hypermagnesaemia in renal failure (weakness, coma, respiratory arrest). Absorption of drugs given concomitantly may be altered.

The commonest problem with intensive antacid regimes is diarrhoea, which may afflict up to half the patients. One recommendation is to make up a mixture of equal parts of magnesium trisilicate BPC and aluminium hydroxide gel BP. This is cheap and has high buffering capacity. If the resulting mixture causes diarrhoea or constipation, the ratio of the constituents can be altered accordingly.

One possible disadvantage of this scheme might be the relatively high sodium content of both constituents. Where sodium load is an important consideration, e.g. in cardiac, renal or hepatic failure or hypertension, Asilone, Mylanta or Maalox might be a better choice. In terms of patient acceptability, of a variety of mixtures tested, Dijex and Mylanta emerged favourably from one study. Dijex is also very cost effective. In general, however, because of the very large volumes involved, intensive antacid regimes are at least as expensive as cimetidine therapy and often more so. The very large volumes required are also socially inconvenient. It is frequently stated that British patients would be unlikely to tolerate the large volumes, in contradistinction to their American counterparts. The author has used these regimes on occasion and has encountered no particular problem with compliance.

Other Treatments

Tricyclics

The tricyclic antidepressant drugs have been shown to be effective in reducing histamine-stimulated secretion of acid and pepsin by the stomach. Trimipramine has also been investigated. The inhibitory effect is dose-related. The mechanism is not clear, but it may be partly explained by the drug's anticholinergic effects.

Clinical trials have repeatedly shown trimipramine to be effective in promoting the healing of duodenal ulcers. Fifty milligrams at night is an effective dose, but causes appreciable drowsiness; 25 mg alone is not an effective dose, but combining this with 120 ml antacid (neutralising capacity 480 mmol) causes ulcer healing with few side-effects.

Pirenzepine is a tricyclic, but it differs from others in the group in that the molecule is hydrophilic. This means that it has very limited capacity to penetrate the blood-brain barrier. Thus the drug is virtually free of CNS side-effects but is a potent inhibitor of gastric secretion. In daily dosage ranging from 75 to 150 mg the drug has been shown in several double-blind controlled studies to be effective in accelerating healing of duodenal ulcers. It appears to be as effective as cimetidine. Side-effects are few, but include dry mouth and double vision.

Prostaglandins

Prostaglandins of the A and E classes are potent antisecretory agents when given intravenously. The natural prostaglandins are not orally effective due to intragastric dehydrogenation at the C_{15} position. Therefore, to avoid inactivation, PGE_2 analogues have been synthesised which contain methyl groups at the C_{15} or C_{16} position. 15-Methyl PGE_2 and 16,16-di-ethyl PGE_2 have been shown to be effective in inhibiting histamine- and meal-stimulated secretion of acid and pepsin and in suppressing gastrin release in response to a meal. Preliminary clinical trials indicate that this group of drugs is effective in healing duodenal ulcers. The mechanism is not entirely clear and may be related to the 'cytoprotective' effect of prostaglandins.

Metoclopramide

Some studies suggest that metoclopramide is effective in healing duodenal ulcers. Further work is required before these could be recommended for routine clinical use.

Gastrointestinal Hormones

Several gastrointestinal hormones are under study for any ulcer-healing effect they or their derivatives may possess. These include secretin, irogastrone and somatostatin.

Drugs of Uncertain Efficacy

Further studies are needed to assess the efficacy of deglycyrrhizinised liquorice (Caved S) and Proglyarmide.

Drugs which have been claimed to promote duodenal ulcer healing but which are probably ineffective include amylopectin sulphate (Depepsen), geranyl farnesylacetate (gefarnate) and prindamine.

Maintenance Therapy

It has become clear that none of the drugs at present available "cure" the underlying disease. That is to say, on stopping therapy, duodenal ulcers recur rapidly. This phenomenon has been best studied with cimetidine.

Cimetidine

Ulcers healed with cimetidine therapy will remain healed if a small dose of the drug is given continuously—usually 400 mg at night. Thus combined results of maintenance trials at 22 centres show that in placebo-treated patients the relapse rate of duodenal ulceration (both symptomatic and clinically silent—detected endoscopically) is approximately 8.5% per month, compared with 2.5% per month with maintenance therapy. After a year's maintenance therapy, the relapse rate on stopping the drug is identical to that after a short course. This seems to be true also after 2 years' maintenance. Thus there is no evidence that cimetidine alters favourably the natural history of the disease. In fact, some authorities suggest that this may be worsened. The integrated gastrin response to a test meal may be increased three-fold after a year's cimetidine. This is not associated with an increase in the parietal cell mass or with the number of gastrin-producing cells (G-cells) in the antrum. The effect is, therefore, probably due to increased activity of individual G-cells following a prolonged period of hypochlorhydria. These observations may explain the occasional reports of perforations occurring following cessation of cimetidine therapy.

Also relevant to the failure of cimetidine to improve the natural history of the disease is the drug's poor effect in restoring the ultrastructural integrity of the duodenal mucosa (compared with De-Nol). Furthermore, cimetidine is reported to have a deleterious effect on gastric mucus. Following cimetidine therapy, the 'cytoprotective index' of gastric mucus is reduced. By contrast this index is raised by carbenoxolone. When the two drugs are combined, cimetidine abolishes the beneficial effect of carbenoxolone. Pirenzepine has no effect on this index.

Duodenal ulceration in many patients is a self-limiting disease in which the symptoms reach a peak some 5–10 years after their onset and then diminish. About two-thirds of patients are asymptomatic or only mildly inconvenienced by dyspepsia 13 years after diagnosis (about 16% come to laparotomy). The question which cannot be answered for many years is this: "Does maintenance cimetidine permit the patient to remain safe and reasonably comfortable whilst the disease goes into spontaneous remission, or is that remission deferred by drug therapy?" What is known is that continuous prophylactic therapy with cimetidine appears safe and effective for periods of up to 2 years. Dosage of 400 mg twice daily confers little if any benefit over 400 mg at night.

Thus, most duodenal ulcers can be healed within 4–6 weeks by cimetidine in a dosage of 1 g daily or 400 mg twice daily. The remainder will mostly heal with more prolonged therapy and/or higher dosage. After healing, relapse is common, most patients suffering one, two or three relapses a year. About 50% of these relapses are asymptomatic, at least initially.

Patients who relapse may be treated with intermittent courses of cimetidine in full dosage. On the other hand, relapses can largely be prevented by maintenance therapy of 400 mg cimetidine at night. Patients who fail to heal or who relapse frequently can be sent for surgery. Each of these treatment options will be considered in turn.

Intermittent Courses of Cimetidine

With this approach, relapses are treated symptomatically (although endoscopy may be used to confirm the presence of an ulcer crater), with standard courses of therapy.

The advantages include:

1. With a well-defined association between symptoms and therapy, the patient is likely to be motivated and compliance high.

2. This strategy is cheaper than continuous maintenance therapy.

3. The patient's disease is monitored, so that patients who continually relapse can be selected for maintenance therapy or surgery. By the same token, if the disease remits, unnecessary medication is not given.

4. The unknown dangers of continuous therapy are avoided.

The disadvantage is that recurrences of duodenal ulceration are frequently asymptomatic. The risk associated with a 'silent' relapse is unknown. However, amongst patients who present with acute upper gastrointestinal haemorrhage from a duodenal ulcer, around 10% have no significant previous history of dyspepsia. Similarly, duodenal ulcers which perforate are stated to be previously clinically 'silent' in 17%–25% of cases. Thus the patient can only be considered free from risk of these complications if no ulcer crater exists.

Regular endoscopies could be performed on asymptomatic patients but this would be impractical outside major centres.

Continuous Prophylaxis

The advantage of this strategy is that it keeps the maximum number of patients ulcer-free at any given time. The disadvantages are that it is expensive and exposes the patient to the unknown risks of long-term therapy. Furthermore, the therapy does not guarantee freedom from relapse. At the end of 12 months, approximately 15% of patients will have relapsed on maintenance therapy. Data on longer periods are scarce, but a further relapse rate of 10%–12% over the next 12 months has been suggested. Thus cimetidine would appear to be delaying relapses rather than truly preventing them. However, most relapses will respond to a further course of cimetidine in full dosage.

Surgery

All surgery for duodenal ulcer necessarily carries morbidity and mortality. Peri-operative mortality in collected series of elective operations is usually 1% and may be even higher. All operations are irreversible. Even highly selective vagotomy, arguably the operation which interferes least with gastric physiology, is associated with significant side-effects. The most common of these is postprandial distension, which may occur in as many as one-third of cases. Heartburn, nausea, vomiting and diarrhoea and both early and late "dumping" may occur. Also, there is a significant recurrence rate of about 7% after 5–10 years' follow-up. However, a satisfactory outcome can be expected in about 90% of cases.

In summary, highly selective vagotomy is probably the most popular operation for duodenal ulceration. Its success is partly due to its minimal interference with normal gastric function. There is, however, an unknown risk of metabolic complications and carcinoma development. These problems are only now becoming clear with respect to operations which previously enjoyed popularity for duodenal ulceration. Surgery for benign peptic ulcer disease has been reported to be associated with a reduction of life expectancy amounting to 8–9 years.

The situation as regards gastric operations for duodenal ulceration is well summarised by Dr. Ken Wormsley (*Duodenal Ulcer*, Volume 2, Annual research reviews series. Editor D. F. Horrobin, Churchill Livingstone), who invites us to:

. . . imagine the introduction of a new anti-ulcer drug, which kills up to 1% of patients soon after the start of treatment; is associated with at least a 10% rate of overt recurrence of ulceration during the course of treatment; paralyses the stomach, with all the disabling consequences, including postcibal fullness, diarrhoea and dumping; results in anaemia, osteomalacia and gastric cancer in a proportion of patients treated for a few years; and is assessed—not by serial endoscopic examination—but by asking the treated patient how he feels and considering the treatment a failure only if the patient is fairly severely disabled. Everyone is allowed to (and does) use the drug, without any check or audit.

Choice of Treatment

One of the most characteristic features of duodenal ulcer disease is the way in which symptoms occur episodically over many years. A majority of patients can be kept comfortable by treating symptomatic relapses by intermittent courses of therapy, usually cimetidine. If this fails to produce symptomatic relief, one might switch to De-Nol, intensive antacid therapy, carbenoxolone or pirenzepine. Many clinicians would be prepared to be guided by symptoms and not to require repeated endoscopies to check for healing or to discover asymptomatic relapses. However, this will depend on personal philosophy and local resources.

Patients who have severe symptoms and who relapse promptly and repeatedly when medication ceases should be considered for either long-term prophylactic cimetidine or surgery. Medical therapy is obviously justified in patients who are elderly or whose general state precludes operation. Young fit patients form a difficult group. It may be wise to discuss the options available with the patient. Some patients are anxious to avoid operation if at all possible. Others will prefer a definitive procedure to an uncertain future with continued consumption of tablets. A good proportion will look for firm guidance from their medical adviser. The author is in favour of prophylactic therapy. This is because the long-term effects of surgery and maintenance cimetidine are both unknown, but the latter is at least reversible.

In practical terms, operation rates have fallen sharply since the advent of cimetidine. Many felt that this would be a temporary phenomenon. There is, however, no evidence of a "catching up" acceleration of operation rates.

Many surgeons are concerned that patients now being referred to them are different than before. These are patients who have responded poorly or incompletely to cimetidine, and surgeons have been concerned that this group would do poorly with operations designed to reduce acid secretion. The evidence suggests that surgery fares no better or worse than in the pre-cimetidine era.

Thus there is a deep division of opinion as to what constitutes "failure of medical therapy" as an indication for surgery. However, complications remain a prime indication for surgical intervention.

Management of Complications

Perforation

Perforation rates have fallen since the early 1950s. This complication now occurs more commonly in elderly patients than previously, especially in women. In Scotland, perforations occur most frequently between 8 and 10 p.m. on Fridays or Saturdays during January. The relationship, if any, to New Year festivities is uncertain.

Treatment is essentially surgical, with closure of the perforation, often combined with an ulcer-healing procedure, although it may be best to defer the latter procedure if the patient is ill, if there is extensive peritoneal soiling or if the surgeon is inexperienced.

Bleeding

Bleeding from duodenal ulcer causes 12%–38% of cases of bleeding from the upper alimentary tract and accounts for 20% of patients dying from upper alimentary haemorrhage. More than half the patients with bleeding duodenal ulcers are over 60 years of age.

The advent of flexible fibre-optic gastroscopy has led to a reappraisal of the importance of duodenal ulceration as a cause of upper gastrointestinal haemorrhage. In one study, a duodenal ulcer was found in 35% of patients but it was the source of bleeding in only 24%. The remaining patients were bleeding from associated gastric or oesophageal lesions. Thus upper gastrointestinal endoscopy should probably be the initial investigation. Barium radiology should not be performed because:

1. The diagnostic yield is poorer than that of upper gastrointestinal endoscopy.

2. Although an ulcer may be demonstrated radiologically, only infrequently can it be demonstrated convincingly as the source of bleeding.

3. Barium in the intestine precludes the use of arteriography.

In-patient mortality from acute gastrointestinal haemorrhage has remained constant at around 8% ever since the prognosis was improved by the provision of blood transfusion. Thus there is no evidence that the improved diagnosis afforded by endoscopy has been translated into improved management. This has led to the comment that the management must be wrong. There may, however, be a hidden improvement, in that there has been a steady increase in the age of patients admitted with acute gastrointestinal haemorrhage.

The patients who are most at risk of dying are the elderly, those who have suffered a severe haemorrhage, those bleeding from a chronic gastric ulcer or oesophageal varices and, most especially, those with recurrent haemorrhage. Thus efforts should be made to identify this high-risk group, as these should certainly be carefully monitored and they may benefit from early surgery.

The greatest risk of rebleeding occurs within 48 h of the initial bleed. After 3 days there is little if any risk of further rebleeding if the initial bleeding was mild (haemoglobin greater than 9 g/100 ml). Rebleeding is most common where the initial bleed is severe. One indication of this is haematemesis, which is usually associated with a loss of more than one-quarter of the circulating red cell volume (melaena alone indicates a smaller bleed).

Patients should be admitted to hospital, preferably to an intensive care unit. Care is best undertaken by a joint medical and surgical team. Measurement of central venous pressure (CVP) is of benefit for the following reasons:

1. CVP monitoring permits rapid and safe re-expansion of blood volume by transfusion, and this gives a measure of initial blood loss. Without measurement of CVP transfusion requirements tend to be underestimated.

2. CVP monitoring gives the earliest indication of rebleeding. This has been shown to be much more sensitive than monitoring pulse and blood pressure.

3. If bleeding continues, rapid transfusion can be maintained, if necessary with a pump, without overloading the heart, so that the patient goes to theatre with a normal blood volume.

Measurement of arterial blood pH is also advantageous as major haemorrhage is frequently associated with an acidosis, which should be corrected.

In the case of a major bleed, endoscopy should be performed as soon as the patient has been resuscitated. If the stomach is full of blood so that the bleeding site is not identified, it should be washed out with a wide-bore tube and a further endoscopy performed.

A duodenal ulcer may be observed to be actively bleeding. Arterial blood may be seen spurting out in an obviously pulsatile way. Alternatively, capillary blood may ooze from the ulcer. If bleeding has stopped, fresh clot will be seen in the base of the ulcer. Localised fresh clot often lies on an arterial bleeding site—"the visible vessel". This appearance is associated with an increased risk of re-bleeding.

Cautery to a bleeding site or visible vessel has been applied via the endoscope, using lasers, diathermy or heater probes. None of these has been fully evaluated clinically, apart from the low-powered Argon laser which seems ineffective in controlling clinically significant bleeding. However, the more powerful Neodinium Yag laser may be more effective.

Arteriography may be valuable in identifying the site of bleeding, especially if endoscopy has failed to do so. The technique will only succeed in the presence of active bleeding—hence the value of a CVP line to detect recurrent or continuing haemorrhage. As well as showing where bleeding is coming from, therapeutic manoeuvres may be tried, such as the infusion of vasoconstrictors or embolisation of a bleeding vessel.

Whilst interventional radiology and endoscopy are of great interest in specialised units, severe or recurrent bleeding will normally be dealt with surgically.

There is no evidence that cimetidine reduces haemorrhage from an acutely bleeding duodenal ulcer. However, many clinicians will start therapy with cimetidine when a duodenal ulcer is found in order to accelerate healing.

There are conflicting reports as to the efficacy of infusions of tranexamic acid in reducing continuing or recurrent haemorrhage in patients with bleeding from the upper gastrointestinal tract. Optimistic results have been reported with infusions of somatostatin. Both forms of therapy warrant further investigation, but neither can be recommended for routine use.

Pyloric Stenosis

This is dealt with surgically, although the author has encountered a few patients with severe symptoms and signs of pyloric stenosis who settled completely with cimetidine, presumably by reduction of spasm and oedema. Thus a trial of medical therapy may be warranted.

Gastric Ulcer

Pathophysiology

Gastric ulceration will be considered separately from duodenal ulceration. On the face of it, this separation appears easy. Duodenal ulceration can be defined as occurring distal to the pyloric ring in intestinal mucosa, whilst gastric ulcers lie proximal to the pylorus in gastric mucosa. Patients with duodenal ulcers have basal and stimulated levels of gastric acid and pepsin which are, on average, greater than levels in normal subjects. By contrast, levels tend to be lower than normal in patients harbouring gastric ulcers. Thus duodenal ulcer may be due to an excessive acid attack on relatively healthy mucosa, whereas gastric ulcer may develop in an unhealthy mucosa that succumbs to a reduced acid attack. Ulcers tend to breed "true". There is an increased incidence of peptic ulcers in the relatives of patients with an ulcer. This increased incidence is almost entirely due to duodenal ulcer if the index case has a duodenal ulcer. Likewise, gastric ulcers are clustered within affected families. The same trend emerges from twin studies. Blood group O non-secretor status is much more strongly linked to duodenal ulceration than to gastric ulceration; indeed, ulcer of the gastric body is rather commoner in patients of blood group A. The diseases have quite different geographical distributions. Gastric ulcers occur on average later in life than duodenal ulcers.

On closer inspection, this distinction is less easily made. All descriptions of chronic peptic ulcer sites show a continuous band extending from the upper gastric lesser curve down to the angulus, along the roof of the antrum and through the pylorus into the duodenal bulb and beyond, with concentrations near the gastric angulus and the first part of the duodenum. There is not always a clear-cut junction between gastric and duodenal mucosa coinciding exactly with the pylorus. Duodenal mucosa may encroach 2 cm proximal to the pylorus, with Brunner's glands extending into the antrum. Alternatively, gastric mucosa, including parietal cells, may extend distal to the pylorus, and this seems to occur especially in the presence of a duodenal ulcer. The site of gastric ulcers has been related to the junction between alkali-secreting and acid-secreting mucosa. The antral mucosa in gastric ulcer tends to show features of chronic atrophic gastritis and intestinal metaplasia. With ulcers high in the stomach, the alkali-secreting area is large, with consequent diminution of the parietal cell area and reducing acid output. Distal gastric ulcer, on the other hand, is associated with a low junction, increased parietal cell mass, and a normal or raised acid output. Thus gastric ulcers occurring near the pylorus behave much more like duodenal ulcers, and this has led many authorities to classify them separately as 'pre-pyloric' or 'juxta-pyloric' ulcers. Unfortunately, because of the continuous distribution of ulcers, it is not feasible to make a precise separation. Another difficulty concerns the fairly large group of patients in whom gastric and duodenal ulcers coexist. In these patients the duodenal ulcer is thought always to precede the gastric ulcer, and acid secretion tends to be high. There is often evidence of gastric outflow obstruction.

Thus it may be more realistic to divide peptic ulcers into four groups:

1. "True" gastric ulcers—occurring high in the body of the stomach, associated with extensive atrophic gastritis and low basal and stimulated gastric acid secretion. This lesion probably results from impaired mucosal resistance to acid. Bile reflux and/or impaired mucus secretion may be important in this respect.

2. "True" duodenal ulceration.

3. Combined gastric and duodenal ulceration (the gastric ulcer probably occurring secondary to duodenal ulcer disease, perhaps due to gastric stasis or bile reflux).

4. Pre-pyloric ulcers occurring within a few centimetres of the pylorus on the gastric side.

Types 2, 3 and 4 all tend to be associated with high basal and stimulated gastric acid secretion.

From a practical standpoint, although it seems likely that these various types of gastric ulcer will respond differently to the various therapeutic manoeuvres, there has been little systematic study on the point. Some series exclude pre-pyloric and combined ulcers; others lump all ulcers occurring between cardia and pylorus in together. Furthermore, drugs effective against duodenal ulcer are often considered active against gastric ulceration as well.

Diagnosis

The whole management of gastric ulcer is dominated by the risk that there may be coexistent malignancy. It is wise to regard any ulcer in the stomach as potentially malignant. It is not possible on clinical grounds accurately to distinguish gastric from duodenal ulceration, nor benign from malignant gastric ulceration. Thus it is essential that patients suspected of having a peptic ulcer should be fully investigated. The choice between endoscopy and barium radiology as the initial investigation depends largely on local circumstances. In this context, a single-contrast barium meal is a waste of time. A well-conducted double-contrast examination will give comparable accuracy to an endoscopy in discovering a peptic ulcer. However, all gastric ulcers must be submitted to endoscopic biopsy and cytological examination. This is because neither radiology nor inspection of a gastric ulcer at endoscopy can reliably exclude malignancy. Multiple (at least six) biopsies must be taken around the edge of the ulcer crater, from the base and from any suspicious adjacent fold.

Endoscopy with biopsy and cytology should be repeated at monthly intervals until complete healing has occurred. The ulcer scar should be biopsied. Failure to heal is an indication for surgery.

Treatment

General Measures

In 1964 Richard Doll made his famous statement that "gastric ulcer is one of the few conditions which provide an opportunity for practising 19th century medicine in the second half of the 20th". This should no longer be true, and this is largely due to Doll himself, who in a classic series of papers laid the foundations for modern therapy.

Diet

Doll showed that none of the diets suggested for patients with gastric ulcer had any effect in accelerating healing. He also showed that a milk drip, with or without added alkali, was ineffective in healing gastric ulcers, although pain was more rapidly relieved and patients gained weight.

Bed Rest

He showed that gastric ulcers healed more rapidly when patients were treated as hospital in-patients with enforced bed rest.

Cigarette Smoking

He confirmed that gastric ulcers were commoner in cigarette smokers and showed that healing was accelerated when the habit was stopped.

Drug Treatment

Doll also showed in two clinical trials that carbenoxolone was an effective agent in healing gastric ulcers. He was limited by the technology of the time. Ulcer healing was assessed by reduction in size of gastric ulcers demonstrated in profile using a single-contrast barium meal technique. This would no longer be regarded as adequate, but few of Doll's experiments have been repeated adequately with endoscopic monitoring. Generally speaking, gastric ulcer has been more poorly investigated than duodenal ulceration. Gastric ulcers are less common than duodenal ulcers, and the prevalence of both lesions has fallen since the early 1950s. Gastric ulcer also affects an older age group than duodenal ulcers, so the patients may be more difficult to investigate. Both duodenal and gastric ulcers have a high placebo healing rate which makes them difficult to study because large groups are necessary.

Schwartz in 1910 enunciated the dictum "no acid—no ulcer". Patients with gastric ulcer on average have lower basal and stimulated gastric acid secretion than normal. However, there are only a handful of cases in the literature where ulcers have occurred in a stomach which demonstrates histamine-fast achlorhydria (interestingly, in some of these rare cases there is a history of high aspirin intake, so it is possible that these cases form a separate group.) The conventional model of an ulcer postulates a balance between acid and pepsin attack and mucosal defence. The mucosa in a stomach containing an ulcer is usually abnormal, showing a variable degree of chronic atrophic gastritis. It is thought that this change renders the mucosa more vulnerable to acid attack— although at the same time the parietal cell mass is diminished and acid output falls (in addition, hydrogen ion may leak out of the stomach more readily than normal). It appears, however, that if acid output can be brought sufficiently low, even impaired mucosal defences will be capable of preventing ulcer formation.

Antacids

There is no definitive trial which demonstrates benefit from antacids in gastric ulcer. In fact, the only double-blind, endoscopically monitored, controlled trial to show benefit concerned a total of only 16 patients, and was surprising in showing 100% healing after 30 days' treatment.

Nonetheless, it is customary to prescribe antacids for symptomatic relief, although, as with duodenal ulceration, the effect may be no better than that obtained with a placebo.

Cimetidine

Cimetidine appears to be effective in accelerating healing of benign gastric ulceration. Thus pooling the results of four trials involving 185 patients showed 60%–80% of ulcers healing, compared with 37%–57% on placebo. American trials showed less clear-cut results, but this may be related to the large amounts of antacid given in the placebo groups. Indeed, a large multicentre trial involving 206 patients showed no significant difference between cimetidine therapy and a median daily antacid consumption of 328 mEq. These data are difficult to interpret until the precise benefit of antacid therapy has been defined.

Carbenoxolone

As previously noted, carbenoxolone was the first drug convincingly demonstrated to have a beneficial effect in gastric ulcer. The drug, derived from liquorice, has been shown to diminish the abnormally raised cell turnover rate in atrophic gastritis and to promote secretion of mucus. Thus the drug probably operates through increasing mucosal resistance to acid attack. Combination therapy with carbenoxolone and cimetidine would therefore appear rational and has indeed been found to be effective.

The sodium- and water-retaining and potassium-losing effects of carbenoxolone have been mentioned (see "Duodenal Ulceration"). Spironolactone reverses these effects, but also antagonises the gastric ulcer-healing properties of the drug and is thus contra-indicated. The mechanism for this effect is unknown, although spironolactone frequently causes gastrointestinal upsets and gastric ulceration apparently caused by the drug has occasionally been reported. Carbenoxolone remains effective in gastric ulceration if patients are simultaneously treated with thiazide. However, thiazide diuretics potentiate potassium loss and treatment must be carefully monitored. There is some suggestion that amiloride may also interfere with the ulcer-healing effect of carbenoxolone.

Several studies have been published comparing carbenoxolone and cimetidine treatment for gastric ulceration. No difference has been shown between the two drugs in terms of efficacy, although side-effects are commoner with carbenoxolone. As the majority of patients with gastric ulceration are over 60 years of age, cimetidine is the drug of choice.

Comparisons of drugs in gastric ulcer are difficult to perform and interpret. Very large numbers of patients will be required to demonstrate a small but possibly important difference. Take the case of a comparison between two drugs, one capable of healing 80% of ulcers and the other 70% in a given time scale. In order to have a reasonable (90%) chance of demonstrating a difference significant at the 5% level, it is easy to calculate that one would need more than 300 patients with gastric ulceration *on each drug*. None of the published comparative series is of anywhere near this size.

Other Drugs

Reports of successful trials in healing gastric ulcers have been reported with De-Nol, trimipramine and pirenzepine. Probably ineffective drugs include metoclopramide and gefarnate.

Besides their anti-secretory effects, PGE_2 derivatives have been shown to increase the thickness of the gastric mucus coat and are, therefore, promising agents in gastric ulceration.

Maintenance Therapy

Gastric ulcers frequently relapse after successful healing—probably around 40% after 12 months. The relapse rate may be slightly less after carbenoxolone than after cimetidine. Cimetidine is probably effective in preventing relapse, although the evidence on this point is incomplete.

Management of Complications

Bleeding

Bleeding gastric ulcers carry a high mortality, and continuing or recurrent haemorrhage should normally be an indication for surgery. Suggestions that cimetidine was helpful in treating bleeding in elderly patients with gastric ulcer have not been substantiated. Somatostatin may be more helpful. Interventional radiological or endoscopic procedures are under study but are not of proven benefit (see "Duodenal Ulceration").

Perforation

Perforation of gastric ulcers is fortunately rare. In one series of 242 perforated peptic ulcers, one fifth occurred in gastric lesions. Treatment is surgical.

Hourglass Stomach

Progressive fibrosis in association with a chronic gastric ulcer may lead to constriction of the mid-portion of the stomach—the hourglass deformity. It is fortunately rare and becoming rarer. Treatment is surgical.

Surgery

Surgical therapy for gastric ulceration is unsatisfactory. Older procedures aimed to remove the ulcer-bearing area of the stomach. The present trend is to more conservative therapy, the object being to reduce acid secretion, usually by means of a selective vagotomy. This is frequently combined with local resection of the ulcer, which makes possible comprehensive histological examination if there is any suspicion of malignancy and also removes the crater itself with the attendant risk of bleeding.

Bleeding gastric ulcers may be treated as above, but often a gastric resection will be needed, especially if the lesion is distal, when a Billroth I procedure may be safer.

Further Reading

Bardhan KD (1981) Perspectives in duodenal ulcer, 2nd edn. Smith Kline and French Laboratories, Philadelphia
Baron JH (ed) (1981) Cimetidine in the 80s. Churchill Livingstone, Edinburgh London New York

Baron JH, Langman MJS, Wastell C (1980) Stomach and duodenum. In: Bouchier IAD (ed) Recent advances in gastroenterol, vol 4. Churchill Livingstone, Edinburgh London New York, pp 23–86

Schiller LR, Feldmann M (1981) Medical therapy of peptic ulcer disease. In: Baron JH, Moody FG (eds) Gastroenterology 1: Foregut. Butterworths International Medical Reviews. Butterworth, London, pp 192–240

3 The Malabsorption Syndrome
R. E. Barry

Pathophysiology

Malabsorption is not a disease. It is, however, a common consequence of many disease processes which may affect different parts of the gastrointestinal tract. It is the clinical syndrome which results from failure to absorb food or food constituents.

Food cannot be absorbed until it is digested; thus failure of digestion (for example due to pancreatic exocrine failure) will cause malabsorption.

The three major components of diet are carbohydrate, protein and fat. Prior to absorption each is digested, firstly by the action of digestive enzymes, predominantly from the pancreatic juice, in the gastrointestinal lumen. After this luminal phase, digestion is completed by membrane-bound enzymes on the brush border of the intestinal epithelial cell.

Carbohydrate

Carbohydrate is ingested predominantly as amylose and amylopectin but also includes disaccharides—for example, sucrose and lactose. The luminal phase of digestion with pancreatic enzymes (amylase) liberates monosaccharides and oligosaccharides (limit dextrins). Monosaccharides such as glucose are absorbed by a (sodium-dependent) active transport process. Disaccharides and oligosaccharides are adsorbed on to the intestinal brush border, where membrane-bound enzymes complete the digestion to monosaccharides, which are then absorbed by their active transport mechanisms. For example, lactose is hydrolysed to glucose and galactose, which are then absorbed. The products of digestion are delivered to the portal circulation.

Protein

Protein is digested in the luminal phase predominantly by pancreative proteases to free amino acids and oligopeptides. The free amino acids are absorbed by one of four independent and relatively specific transport mechanisms. Oligo-peptides are absorbed onto the intestinal brush border, where membrane-bound enzymes can complete the digestion and the liberated amino acids are absorbed. However, recent work indicates that some di- and tripeptides and perhaps even oligopeptides may be absorbed intact. Other dipeptides may be absorbed into the intestinal epithelial cell and digestion completed intracellu-larly. The products of digestion are absorbed into the portal circulation.

Fat

Fat is ingested as triglyceride. Luminal digestion by pancreatic lipase liberates free fatty acids and β-monoglyceride. These products of fat digestion are not freely water soluble. An additional step is therefore necessary in the digestion/absorption process for fat which is not necessary for carbohydrate or protein absorption. This step involves the solubilisation of the products of triglyceride digestion. The free fatty acids and the β-monoglyceride are taken up into a micellar solution by forming mixed micelles with bile salts. Micelles will only form if the detergent (bile salts) is present in sufficient concentration, i.e. only if "the critical micellar concentration" is exceeded. Free fatty acids and β-monoglycerides are absorbed from the micellar solution into the intestinal cell. Once inside the intestinal cell, the triglyceride is *resynthesised* by the re-esterification of free fatty acid and monoglyceride. This newly formed fat is then "packaged' into particles called chylomicrons in which a central core of triglyceride is enveloped by an outer layer of β-lipoprotein. This particle is then delivered, *not* to the portal circulation but to the lymphatic system, and reaches the systemic circulation via the thoracic duct.

Because luminal digestion and an intact epithelium are essential to the digestion and absorption of protein, carbohydrate and fat, malabsorption of all three food constituents will occur in the presence of pancreatic exocrine failure and also in extensive disturbance of the intestinal epithelial cell function such as occurs in coeliac disease.

However, there are additional steps which are necessary for the absorption of fat (such as micellar solubilisation, intracellular re-esterification, chylomicron formation and also an additional delivery system to the circulation) but are not present in carbohydrate or protein absorption. Consequently there are more points at which fat absorption may be disturbed. As a result, diseases causing malabsorption are most likely to affect fat absorption, rather than carbohydrate or protein, producing steatorrhoea. Because of this, and since fat is relatively easy to measure in stool, the measurement of faecal fat is the most widely used estimate of malabsorption.

Diagnosis

There are two important questions in the diagnosis of malabsorption. Firstly, is malabsorption present? Secondly, what is the disease which is causing the malabsorption? A third question, what is being malabsorbed?, is relevant in treatment but rarely helps diagnosis.

Is Malabsorption Present?

This may be suggested by the clinical history or physical examination. Often certain laboratory findings such as a mixed deficiency anaemia or isolated deficiencies (e.g. of fat soluble vitamins or folic acid) may suggest malabsorption. Although many screening tests have been devised to answer this question, the most reliable and widely used is a faecal fat balance. If the daily faecal fat output exceeds 15 mmol on a 100 g fat diet, then malabsorption of fat is present.

What Is the Disease Causing the Malabsorption?

This question is usually answered by the following two simple investigations. A barium follow-through will reveal gross anatomical abnormalities of the small intestine such as intestinal fistulae, strictures and Crohn's disease. The *mechanism* by which these abnormalities cause the malabsorption is beyond the scope of this book. If the barium follow-through is *normal*, then the second investigation is jejunal biopsy. Histological examination of the microscopic anatomy of the small intestinal mucosa makes possible the diagnosis of many of the remaining causes of malabsorption, such as coeliac disease, giardiasis, abetalipoproteinaemia, lymphangiectasia and sprue.

If both the barium follow-through and the jejunal biopsy are normal in the presence of steatorrhoea, then pancreatic failure is *likely* to be the cause and this can then be confirmed by specific tests of pancreatic exocrine function.

Therapeutic Principles

Aims of Treatment

The primary aim of treatment is, where possible, to correct the malabsorption syndrome by treating the disease which is causing it. For example, coeliac disease is treated with a gluten-free diet and extrahepatic biliary obstruction is treated by surgical relief. Where the disease process is not remediable, an understanding of the mechanisms involved may allow the malabsorption itself to be effectively treated. For example, malabsorption caused by chronic pancreatitis can be cured by oral pancreatic enzyme replacements even though the disease process in the pancreas persists.

In addition, treatment should be directed at the *consequences* of malabsorption. Thus iron and folic acid may be required to correct anaemia or vitamin D to correct osteomalacia, which may be present as a consequence of the malabsorption syndrome.

General Management

Until the malabsorption syndrome is controlled and the patient is nutritionally restored, the diet should be high in calorie and protein content. Because fats exacerbate the symptoms of steatorrhoea, the dietary fat content should be reduced or eliminated as necessary. Medium chain triglyceride is usually well tolerated and can be used as a calorie supplement.

Deficiency of the fat soluble vitamins A, D and K is common. Vitamin A deficiency rarely causes symptoms but can be detected by special investigation. Vitamin D deficiency is particularly common in the United Kingdom, where climate and dietary habits make subclinical osteomalacia relatively common even in the absence of malabsorption. Vitamin D deficiency is by no means unusual as a presenting feature of malabsorption.

Disordered clotting, due to malabsorption of vitamin K, is commonly detectable as a prolonged prothrombin time, but spontaneous bleeding caused by this is unusual except in the very acute or very prolonged (undiagnosed) malabsorptive states.

Oral supplements of vitamin D may suffice in mild malabsorption, but parenteral administration of vitamins D and K are preferable and more predictable in their effect. Doses should be tailored to individual requirements and may need to be large in severe or long-standing steatorrhoea. Phytomenadione 10 mg intramuscularly weekly and calciferol 3000 IU intramuscularly weekly is usually sufficient maintenance treatment for mild to moderate malabsorption in the absence of liver disease. Where osteomalacia is well established, 50 000 IU of calciferol daily plus calcium supplementation may be required (beware of hypercalcaemia). 1α-Hydroxycholecalciferol (converted to 1,25-di-hydroxycholecalciferol) is now available and is rapidly effective but requires frequent monitoring for hypercalcaemia.

Most patients with malabsorption develop folate deficiency. This is so common that red cell folate estimation is sometimes used as a screening test for malabsorption. The deficiency is frequently severe enough to produce a macrocytic anaemia. Unlike dietary folates which are polyglutamates, folic acid tablets (pteroylmonoglutamates) are rapidly absorbed. Consequently oral treatment with folic acid tablets 10 mg three times daily is usually sufficient to correct the anaemia, but accurate diagnosis is essential because malabsorption caused by mucosal disease of the terminal ileum (such as extensive coeliac disease or terminal ileal Crohn's disease) will also cause malabsorption of vitamin B_{12}. In this instance treatment with folic acid will correct the anaemia so that vitamin B_{12} deficiency may remain undiagnosed until irreversible neuropathy develops.

Vitamin B_{12} is stored in the liver and serum vitamin B_{12} deficiency does not occur until these stores have been exhausted, which will take months or even years. The presence of vitamin B_{12} deficiency suggests long-standing ileal disease.

Co-existing vitamin B_{12} deficiency is treated parenterally with hydroxycoba-lamine 1000 μg intramuscularly monthly. Cyanocobalamine should not now be used because of the occasional precipitation of toxic amblyopia in susceptible patients.

Although macrocytic anaemia is the classical anaemia to be associated with malabsorption syndromes, the commonest anaemia is microcytic and due to iron deficiency. Oral iron preparations are often sufficient to correct this anaemia, but in severe malabsorption iron dextran given by deep intramuscular injection is required to correct the anaemia and to replenish the body iron stores.

Specific Management of Malabsorption Syndromes

Malabsorption Caused by Luminal Factors

Pancreatic Enzyme Deficiency

Exocrine pancreatic insufficiency is commonly caused by fibrocystic disease (mucoviscidosis) or chronic pancreatitis, which may be alcohol induced, idiopathic or related to biliary tract disease. Established pancreatic insufficiency causes a severe malabsorption syndrome with gross steatorrhoea and severely affects protein, carbohydrate and fat digestion. Except in the rare cases of isolated obstruction to the pancreatic duct drainage, which may respond to surgical relief, pancreatic damage is usually irreversible. Therapy therefore hinges on oral replacement of pancreatic enzymes. Several preparations are available for oral replacement of pancreatic enzymes. Pancreatin tabs. BP have approximately 25% of the enzyme content of Pancrex V capsules; Pancrex V Forte are enteric coated but actually contain slightly less enzymes per unit weight than Pancrex capsules despite the suffix Forte. Cotazym has a higher lipase content than other preparations. Granular forms of pancreatic extract are also available.

The dose required is that dose which will eliminate or reverse weight loss and correct the steatorrhoea in an individual patient. Pancreatic replacement should be administered *with* meals, although hourly doses have been recommended in resistant patients. Pancreatic replacements should not be sprinkled on hot foods since denaturation will occur.

Pancreatic enzymes have an optimal pH which is *alkaline* and they may therefore be denatured by gastric acid, particularly in the absence of pancreatic bicarbonate secretion. This is why pancreatic enzymes should be taken with food and not before meals. Neutralisation of the gastric acid by antacid mixtures or decreasing the gastric acid output with standard doses of histamine H_2 receptor antagonists such as cimetidine is effective in protecting the pancreatic enzymes from acid destruction, and this treatment should be used in any patient with pancreatic insufficiency who fails to respond clinically to optimal enzyme replacement.

Bile Salt Deficiency

When the concentration of bile salts in the upper small intestine falls below the critical micellar concentration (approximately 2 mM) solubilisation of the products of fat digestion is impaired and steatorrhoea results. This steatorrhoea is maximal in complete biliary obstruction but varying degrees of deficiency occur in acute and chronic hepatic disease (e.g. cirrhosis), where the liver's synthetic capacity is impaired.

Bile salts are reabsorbed from the terminal ileum and are extracted from the serum by the liver for repeat biliary secretion. Consequently, resection or disease of the terminal ileum (e.g. Crohn's disease) causes failure of ileal reabsorption and therefore bile salt wastage. The liver's capacity to compensate for this loss by increased bile salt synthesis may be insufficient and intraluminal bile salt deficiency then results in steatorrhoea.

In chronic liver disease the steatorrhoea is not often of sufficient degree to merit specific therapy. But in complete biliary obstruction the steatorrhoea may be severe and surgical relief is then the treatment of choice. Oral bile salt replacement is impracticable because of its cathartic action and the poor cost effectiveness.

The upper small intestine normally contains fewer than 10^3 bacteria per millilitre of fluid contents. This figure is considerably exceeded in the condition of small bowel bacterial contamination, which occurs in many situations (see below). The abnormal flora in this condition contains many anaerobic bacteria which are capable of deconjugating bile salts. In their unconjugated form bile salts are of little use in fat solubilisation and tend to precipitate at lower pHs. Consequently the concentration of *conjugated* (useful) bile salts may fall below the critical micellar concentration in small bowel bacterial contamination and steatorrhoea may therefore result. Treatment with antibiotics (see below) is the treatment of choice.

Hostile Luminal Environment

There are several factors which may alter the environmental conditions in the gastrointestinal tract and by so doing interfere with digestion or absorption to produce a malabsorption syndrome. As indicated above, an abnormally low duodenal pH such as occurs in Zollinger-Ellison syndrome can denature or precipitate pancreatic enzymes and cause malabsorption. Gastrectomy or treatment with large doses of histamine H_2 receptor antagonists may be effective in correcting this.

Abnormally large bacterial flora in the small intestine can produce malabsorption by the mechanisms discussed above. The factors which normally maintain the relative sterility of the normal small intestine are incompletely understood. Normal gastric acid secretion, normal motility and normal secretion of mucosal immunoglobulin (IgA) appear to be important factors. Disturbances of these protective mechanisms are often associated with varying degrees of small bowel bacterial contamination. Mild degrees of malabsorption can be detected in some elderly patients with achlorhydria.

Disturbed intestinal motility occurring in scleroderma, intestinal strictures, pseudo-obstructive syndromes, ileus etc. is frequently associated with marked malabsorption caused by the associated abnormal flora which develops.

The largest abnormal flora develops in the presence of entero-enteric fistulae. Most of the malabsorption which occurs, for example, in gastrocolic fistulae is caused by the passage of bacteria from the colon to the small intestine via the stomach and not, as popularly supposed, by a short-circuiting effect of food to the colon. Thus many of the symptoms caused by entero-enteric fistulae will respond to appropriate antibiotic treatment.

Solitary large diverticulum of the duodenum is common but rarely supports a sufficiently large flora to produce clinically significant malabsorption. However, multiple small intestinal diverticula can result in a severe malabsorption syndrome due to the flora present in the diverticula. Similarly, surgically created intestinal "blind loops" commonly result in malabsorption.

Malabsorption associated with small bowel bacterial contamination affects predominantly fat absorption secondary to the bacterial effects on bile salts. However, mild mucosal changes can occur. It may be that some mild impairment of carbohydrate and protein absorption may occur secondarily to this mucosal damage, but it is more likely that any such impaired absorption of these two food constituents is likely to be multifactorial in origin. The bacteria also affect small intestinal motility and, indeed, a complete ileus may result from small bowel bacterial contamination.

Vitamin B_{12} malabsorption is common in small bowel bacterial contamination. This is rarely sufficient to cause subacute combined degeneration of the cord but it often produces macrocytic anaemia. The exact mechanism by which the vitamin B_{12} malabsorption occurs has not been well elucidated, but some bacteria undoubtedly bind vitamin B_{12} in the lumen and render it unabsorbable whereas other bacteria can split the vitamin B_{12}–intrinsic factor complex.

The treatment of small bowel bacterial contamination should be directed at the cause, e.g. surgical resection of the strictures or fistulae. Often, however, the cause is not amenable to surgery, e.g. in jejunal diverticulosis. Here, antibiotics play a major role in management. Even where surgery is indicated, a patient's nutrition can often be considerably improved prior to operation by antibiotic treatment, which reduces the flora and corrects the malabsorption.

The choice of antibiotic for use in small bowel bacterial contamination is open to question. Traditional teaching is to use broad spectrum oral antibiotics such as tetracycline over long periods. This is probably unnecessary and potentially dangerous. The risk of superinfection by staphylococci or candida, the frequency of antibiotic-induced diarrhoea and the incidence of the pseudomembranous colitis syndrome would suggest that short courses of narrow spectrum antibiotics are preferable on theoretical grounds. Symptoms will frequently remit within hours, or a day or two, of starting appropriate antibiotic treatment. There is evidence to suggest that the intestinal flora is insensitive to an individual antibiotic within a week of starting treatment. On the other hand, the length of remission following antibiotic treatment, although variable, is often weeks or months despite this. Although some aerobic organisms seem capable of bile salt deconjugation, there is no doubt that anaerobic organisms are quantitatively much more important in producing this effect. It should be remembered that antibiotics can *not* eradicate an enteric flora and that the emergence of antibiotic resistance in an enteric bacterial population is rapid. The aims of treatment therefore are to *change* the flora sufficiently to improve the symptoms by *decreasing* the anaerobic population.

Because of these factors it is preferable to treat the small bowel bacterial contamination syndromes with short courses of narrow spectrum antibiotics which are specifically effective against obligate anaerobes; for example, oral metronidazole 400 mg three times a day for 5 days. A clinical response may be expected within the first days of treatment and is usually maintained after stopping the drug. Unless the cause of bacterial contamination has been eliminated, relapse can be expected after an unpredictable time interval. When this occurs, a repeated course of the *same* antibiotic will frequently produce a similar beneficial effect, so that repeated short courses of the same antibiotic can be administered as and when symptoms indicate. However, experience shows that patients will become symptomatically resistant after three or four courses of such an antibiotic. When this occurs a change to a similar oral preparation effective against anaerobes, e.g. erythromycin, 500 mg four times a day, will then be effective until a further change of antibiotics becomes necessary.

Several months frequently elapse before the symptoms fail to respond to a third change of antibiotic, and the intestinal flora has by then often changed sufficiently to be sensitive to the drug of first choice (metronidazole) again. It is therefore well worthwhile repeating a course of the first antibiotic as a trial at this stage and assessing the clinical response.

There is no doubt that some resistant cases will not respond to this approach, in which instance the traditional treatment with long-term broad spectrum antibiotics such as tetracycline should be tried. However, it is wrong to assume that the mere presence of an abnormal small intestinal flora necessarily means that this flora is causing malabsorption, particularly in diseases such as systemic sclerosis or immune deficiency, where changes in the mucosa or intestinal wall may be the dominant pathophysiological factor. Consequently, the response of the patient to antibiotics should be carefully assessed clinically by the remission of symptoms, such as decrease in stool frequency and anorexia or resolution of steatorrhoea and weight gain. In the absence of such a clinical response the antibiotic should be withdrawn to avoid the complications which the antibiotics themselves may induce.

Intestinal infestations are sometimes associated with malabsorption. Of the many infestations which may rarely be associated with malabsorption, only one commonly produces clinically significant malabsorption in the United Kingdom and this is infestation with the protozoon *Giardia lamblia*.

Giardiasis is more common in patients with immunodeficiency and should always be sought as an easily treatable cause of malabsorption in this heterogeneous group of patients. Diagnosis is achieved by finding the protozoon in jejunal aspirates or biopsy or, less easily, by microscopy of the stool. Metronidazole 1.8 g per day is the drug of choice. The rare resistant cases may respond to tinidazole or mepacrine.

Malabsorption Caused by Abnormal Small Intestinal Mucosa

Sensitivity to Dietary Proteins

Intolerance to protein constituents of wheat flour, soya flour and cow's milk can cause severe damage to the intestinal epithelial cell which results in impaired absorption of all dietary constituents.

By far the commonest of this group of diseases is coeliac disease, and only this disease will be discussed in detail since the principles of management are the same in all diseases in this group.

Patients suffering from coeliac disease are intolerant of gluten. Gluten is the collective name which describes the proteins of the wheat germ. The mechanism by which gluten exerts its toxic effect in susceptible patients is unknown. The toxicity of gluten is known to be present in the gliadin fractions of gluten and these proteins remain toxic even after peptic and tryptic digestion.

In coeliac disease the intestinal epithelial cells are damaged or destroyed as they emerge from the small intestinal crypts. The crypts, which act as the progenitor compartment for the small intestinal mucosa, become considerably hyperplastic in an attempt to compensate for this epithelial cell loss by massive increase in epithelial cell production. This greatly accelerated rate of epithelial cell production and loss acts as a significant drain on the body's nutritional resources. Their constituent proteins and lipids and mineral contents are lost into the intestinal lumen, thus compounding the deficiencies caused by malabsorption of the diet. Indeed, in severe cases, this enteric loss of nutrients may exceed the dietary intake. This explains the often observed phenomenon in which the faecal fat content in severe coeliac disease can exceed the dietary fat intake. In coeliac disease the severity of the malabsorption syndrome does not depend on the severity of the mucosal changes but seems related more to the extent of intestinal involvement, which may vary with time. Thus in the acute malabsorption syndrome caused by coeliac disease, where there is severe diarrhoea and weight loss, mucosal changes are likely to be extensive—from the proximal duodenum to the distal ileum, as indicated by a failure to absorb vitamin B_{12}. But in the mild malabsorption of insidious onset, which is now the commoner presentation of coeliac disease in adults, the mucosal changes may be limited to the duodenum and proximal jejunum only.

The intestinal mucosa will recover completely if all gluten is removed from the diet. However, in some patients the histological recovery may be slow, so that the mucosal architecture may remain abnormal for as long as a year or more following the institution of a gluten-free diet ("slow responders"). In the majority of patients, however, a dramatic symptomatic improvement occurs on dietary gluten withdrawal. This improvement in symptoms may occur within days and usually antedates the biochemical and histological evidence of remission.

For a diet to be free of gluten all foods that contain wheat flour or wheat products need to be excluded. Unfortunately, wheat flour is such a basic food commodity that it is found ubiquitously even in food where there is no reason to suspect its presence. For example, plain potato crisps are gluten free, but in flavoured potato crisps the flavouring is often held on to the crisp with gluten. For these reasons close co-operation between the patient, the doctor and the dietitian is essential for successful treatment.

The gluten-free diet can be achieved by simple omission of all gluten-containing foods. However, those foods in which wheat flour is a basic constituent, such as bread, cakes, pastry etc., can be replaced by identical foods which are baked with gluten-free flour. Gluten-free flour, gluten-free bread and bread mixes etc. are prescribable.

Wheat flour is commonly used as garnishing, e.g. in the batter for fish. Consequently many foods are gluten free in their unprocessed form but not in their processed form. Cheese, fish, meat and cream are examples of gluten-free foods, but cheese spreads, fish in batter or breadcrumbs, sausage and tinned meats, and synthetic creams are not gluten free.

Breakfast cereals made from wheat products are forbidden in the gluten-free diet, but breakfast cereals which are produced from maize, e.g. cornflakes, are allowed.

There are other cereals which are toxic to the small intestinal mucosa in patients with coeliac disease in addition to wheat. Barley is undoubtedly toxic to coeliac patients but is rarely used in western diets. However, barley products are found in certain drinks such as barley water and some home-made beers and also in some coffee substitutes.

The toxicity of oats is disputed. Oats may be a valuable source of fibre in a gluten-free diet and seem to be well tolerated by most patients with coeliac disease. However, a few patients with coeliac disease who seem to respond slowly or incompletely to a gluten-free diet are further improved by the additional withdrawal of oats.

In all patients in whom there is damage to the small intestinal epithelium such as occurs in coeliac disease and also in some patients in whom there is mild or subtle damage to the small intestinal epithelium such as occurs in viral enteritis, a relative deficiency of the membrane-bound enzymes results. Consequently an intolerance of disaccharides such as lactose or sucrose is often found as a secondary but temporary and reversible phenomenon. As a consequence of this a simple gluten-free diet is sometimes insufficient to control the symptoms in the early phase of treatment in some patients with coeliac disease, and the additional exclusion of these disaccharides and their substitution with glucose may be necessary.

It has been suggested that some patients with a very severe and poorly responsive coeliac syndrome require oral zinc supplementation to effect a response to treatment, but the evidence for this is as yet incomplete.

The literature on coeliac disease has led to the belief that patients treated with corticosteroids respond well to this treatment even when gluten is not withdrawn from the diet. The evidence on which this belief is based is insubstantial. Certainly there is some cytological evidence of improvement in patients treated with prednisolone on a normal diet. However, the evidence is fragmentary and the numbers studied very small. Nevertheless, oral prednisolone in therapeutic doses is now in common usage in two situations with coeliac disease. Firstly, in those patients who fail to respond to an apparently strict gluten-free diet. Secondly, in the occasional patients who are very severely ill, perhaps because of late diagnosis or a severe or explosive malabsorption syndrome. Here, the corticosteroids are used as an adjunct to dietary gluten withdrawal.

Tropical Sprue

This is a syndrome of malabsorption of unknown aetiology but which is generally held to be of infective aetiology because of its clinical and epidemiological features.

Changes in the small bowel mucosal architecture in chronic tropical sprue are responsible for the malabsorption in this condition. Small bowel bacterial contamination is also frequently, if not invariably, present in tropical sprue but is probably not the primary abnormality. Furthermore, the bacterial flora which does occur in this condition seems to lack the major anaerobic component which is typical of the blind loop syndrome.

The disease occurs characteristically in residents of temperate zones who visit an endemic tropical area. There are two major regions of the world in which the disease is endemic. One is a broad band covering the northern part of the South American continent and Caribbean and the other extends across the southern part of the Asian continent. Some clinicians believe that two varieties of the disease (corresponding to these two different regions) exist which have somewhat different clinical features, but mucosal malabsorption is the dominant feature of both in the chronic stage.

In the Asian form the patient suffers an acute severe diarrhoeal illness — often simultaneously with others in his party or household. Whereas his fellow sufferers may well recover spontaneously after a brief illness, the patient with tropical sprue enjoys only an incomplete remission before following a progressive downhill course characterised by diarrhoea with steatorrhoea, abdominal distension, anorexia and weight loss, followed by the complications of malabsorption such as anaemia.

Diagnosis is made histologically from the jejunal biopsy in a patient with typical symptoms from an endemic area. There is, however, no characteristic change in the mucosal architecture in tropical sprue. Such changes as do occur are extremely variable. In the chronic stage villous shortening and crypt hypoplasia of varying degrees are seen with lamina propria infiltration with round cells. These changes may be severe, but the completely flat biopsy (total or subtotal villous atrophy) is not usual though it is occasionally seen. This can usually be distinguished from coeliac disease by the experienced histopathologist. *Giardia lamblia* infestation sometimes coexists with tropical sprue.

In the very early stages before mucosal architectural changes occur, a profound malabsorption of folic acid and also vitamin B_{12} occurs, at least in the Asian variety of the disease. At this stage tests of general absorptive function may be normal.

Treatment

Correction of folate deficiency with large doses of oral folic acid and treatment of the vitamin B_{12} deficiency with intramuscular hydroxycobalamine will cure some cases of tropical sprue in the early stages. Histological changes in the small intestinal mucosa will also remit on this treatment.

In long-standing cases, however, folic acid and vitamin B_{12} alone rarely suffice, and antibiotic treatment will be required in addition. Treatment should be continued for at least 6 months.

Sulphonamides were the first antimicrobial treatment to be used successfully in the treatment of tropical sprue, but it seems illogical to use this group of drugs concomitantly with folic acid. Tetracycline is the most widely used drug. Recommended doses for adults are 250 mg four times daily for 4 weeks, followed by 250 mg twice daily for a further 5 months.

A good symptomatic response may be expected within 4–6 weeks. In spite of a good initial response, the long-term follow-up studies in the Caribbean form of the disease have revealed a disturbing incidence (up to 50%) of long-term sequelae of chronic low-grade malabsorption and weight loss.

Whipple's Disease

Although the aetiology of this relatively rare disease is as yet unproven, most workers accept that it very probably results from infection.

Whipple's disease is a multisystem disease predominantly affecting joints, lungs, pleura, heart, peritoneum and gastrointestinal tract. Malabsorption, however, is only a *late* complication of the disease. Affected tissues contain large numbers of macrophages which stain with diastase-resistant periodic acid–Schiff (PAS). Electron microscopy reveals large numbers of bacilliform structures within the macrophages which cause the PAS staining and lend credence to the infective theory of the disease's aetiology. Diagnosis is achieved by recognition of these histological characteristics in biopsy material. Jejunal biopsy is the most commonly used material diagnostically, because of ease, availability and safety.

No single organism has been consistently isolated as a causative factor, even from tissues such as lymph nodes where external contamination, which is bound to complicate per oral biopsy studies, should not occur. This has led to speculation that an immune defect, perhaps in the macrophages, may be responsible for the pathogenesis of the disease. However, although various abnormalities in cellular immune function have been described, the findings are in dispute. Furthermore, many such apparent immune abnormalities cannot be a primary phenomenon since they tend to become normal when the disease is successfully treated.

The histological changes on jejunal biopsy are characteristic. In addition to the changes described in the lamina propria, changes occur in the mucosal architecture so that villi become shortened and clubbed. But a "flat" mucosa (total or subtotal villous atrophy) is rare except in occasional small patches. This decrease in surface area may account for some of the accompanying malabsorption which is the characteristic late manifestation of the disease, but exudation from distended lacteals produces additional losses. Thus a protein-losing enteropathy commonly occurs in Whipple's disease, as in other small intestinal mucosal malabsorptive states such as coeliac disease or lymphangiectasia.

Treatment

Whipple's disease is successfully treated by antibiotics. The choice of antibiotic does not seem to be critical and a variety of antibiotics have been used, such as streptomycin, tetracycline, penicillin, erythromycin and sulphonamides. Since such a large variety of drugs have been used successfully, general principles would indicate that the choice of antibiotic should be influenced by safety, cost and patient acceptability. Treatment failures, however, do occur with any single antibiotic but a change to a second drug, e.g. from penicillin to erythromycin, will usually be effective. Broad spectrum antibiotics such as tetracycline have previously been recommended but there is no evidence of an increased cure rate with this group of antimicrobials. There is general agreement, however, that a course of treatment should extend over a minimum period of 1 year and, for this reason at least, the narrower spectrum antibiotics are preferable. Symptomatic response occurs very early in the course of treatment. The end point for treatment is established histologically, again using jejunal biopsy tissue. Treatment ends when the patient is symptom free, after a minimum of 1 year, provided that all PAS-positive macrophages have disappeared from the lamina propria. But relapses after apparently successful treatment are common and necessitate a further course of antibiotic therapy.

Relapse of central nervous system disease in the absence of gastrointestinal disease has been described, which may perhaps be taken to indicate that the chosen antibiotic should be able to penetrate the blood-brain barrier.

Common Variable Immune Deficiency (Hypogammaglobulinaemia)

This condition of unknown aetiology is associated with malabsorption only in a proportion of cases. Jejunal biopsy may reveal a variety of small intestinal mucosal architectural changes which are sometimes severe enough to mimic the "flat" biopsy of coeliac disease. Often, however, the changes are those of a severe but partial villous atrophy. Immunofluorescent staining of the jejunal mucosa reveals an absence or severe diminution in the numbers of immunoglobulin-producing cells in the lamina propria. This may be the only histological abnormality.

Treatment

A few cases will respond to a gluten-free diet and these cases may arguably represent patients with coexisting coeliac disease. A further proportion of patients will improve symptomatically if treated by weekly replacement injections of gamma-globulin intramuscularly.

Antibiotic therapy has no beneficial effect on the malabsorption but is often indicated for the other consequences of the immune defect, e.g. chronic respiratory infections of bronchiectasis.

However, a careful search for *Giardia lamblia* in jejunal biopsies, small intestinal aspirates or stool is well worthwhile since the incidence of infestation is higher than in the normal population and in affected patients treatment of the giardiasis is often curative of the symptoms.

Dermatitis Herpetiformis

Approximately two-thirds of patients with dermatitis herpetiformis have a mild malabsorption syndrome which can be detected by the usual investigations. But less than half of these patients have symptoms referable to this. Jejunal biopsy in these patients reveals mucosal architectural changes which are indistinguishable from those of coeliac disease except that the changes tend to be more patchy and less severe than those seen in typical untreated coeliac disease. The gastrointestinal symptoms and mucosal changes respond well to treatment with a gluten-free diet. Most gastroenterologists regard coeliac disease and dermatitis herpetiformis as the same disease as far as the gastrointestinal tract is concerned. Patients with dermatitis herpetiformis appear to suffer identical complications (such as lymphoma) to patients with coeliac disease.

Other Mucosal Diseases

Amyloidosis, abetalipoproteinaemia, intestinal lymphangiectasia and other conditions are readily diagnosed on jejunal biopsy. Treatment follows the general principles of management of malabsorption in these conditions, in which no specific therapy exists.

Further Reading

Cooke WT, Asquith P (eds) (1974) Coeliac disease. Clin Gastroenterol 3(1) Saunders, London Philadelphia Toronto
Creamer B (ed) (1974) The small intestine. Heinemann Medical, London
Heaton KW (1972) Bile salts in health and disease. Churchill Livingstone, Edinburgh London New York
Losowsky MS, Walker BE, Kelleher J (1974) Malabsorption in clinical practice. Churchill Livingstone, Edinburgh London New York

4 Infective Diarrhoea

R. E. Barry

Pathophysiology

Infective diarrhoea is a very common medical problem. Although acute diarrhoea is a relatively frequent cause of hospital admission, these patients represent only a small proportion of the cases occurring in a community. Most cases do not require admission since the disease is largely self-limiting and usually brief.

The aetiology of infective diarrhoea varies considerably according to the patient's age and the geographical location. The infective diarrhoeas found in tropical regions are dealt with elsewhere in this book.

In the infective diarrhoeas of childhood, an aetiological agent can be identified in more than 80% of cases. Most of these are viral, with rotavirus being the commonest. Amongst adults, however, an aetiological agent can be found in only a quarter to a third of cases and the large majority of these are bacterial rather than viral in aetiology. The diagnostic success rate has now risen to over 60% (in one recent survey in north-west London), largely because of the more frequent recognition in recent years of two important pathogens: *Clostridium difficile*, which is discussed elsewhere in this volume, and *Campylobacter* species. Even so, in 40% of the diarrhoeas in adults, presumed to be infective, no aetiological agent can be isolated.

The mechanisms by which infective agents produce diarrhoea have only recently begun to be investigated and our knowledge in this vital area is hopelessly incomplete. However, the bacterial diarrhoeas can be roughly classified into two main groups.

Firstly, those caused by invasive organisms which can not only penetrate the gastrointestinal epithelium to produce destructive lesions in the gastrointestinal tract itself, such as ulcers, but also disseminate to cause septicaemia and distant foci of infection. Such an organism is typified by *Salmonella typhi*.

The second group of organisms is typified by *Vibrio cholerae*. Here the diarrhoea is caused by an enterotoxin, secreted by the organism, which attaches to the gastrointestinal epithelium and thereby causes secretion of water and electrolytes into the gastrointestinal tract. But the capacity of the organism to invade the mucosa is absent or virtually so. It is in this latter group of "toxigenic" diarrhoeas where some insight into the pathogenic mechanisms is developing (see below).

This classification is clearly too simplistic. Many organisms, for example many species of *Staphylococcus* or *Salmonella*, can produce enterotoxins and also possess some invasive potential. The relative importance of invasiveness, toxin production and virulence as against that of host defence mechanisms (such as the immune defence mechanisms of the gastrointestinal tract), motility and endogenous and exogenous antibacterial factors has not been studied and may well vary considerably between different patients and different infecting organisms. Consequently the same dose of an infecting organism may produce a clinical illness of widely differing severity in different patients. Nevertheless, this rough classification into invasive or toxigenic organisms is relevant to the management of infective diarrhoea. Clearly, invasive organisms such as *Salmonella typhi* should be treated promptly with full doses of the appropriate antibiotic, whereas in diarrhoea caused by non-invasive toxin-producing organisms antibiotics are often unnecessary and *may even be contra-indicated*.

Cholera is the classic example of a non-invasive enterotoxin-producing organism. After ingestion of an infective dose of cholera vibrios the organism multiplies in the gastrointestinal tract and produces the cholera enterotoxin. This enterotoxin binds rapidly and probably irreversibly with the epithelial cells of the intestine, where it remains for the lifetime of the cell. No structural damage to the epithelial cell is visible. However, the cholera enterotoxin activates plasma membrane-bound adenylate cyclase, probably by transferring ADP-ribose from nicotinamide adenine dinucleotide to a regulatory protein of adenylate cyclase. The activation of adenylate cyclase catalyses the formation of cyclic adenosine 5'-monophosphate (cAMP). This intracellular messenger is able to "switch on" the metabolic processes in the cell, resulting in the secretion of electrolytes into the small intestinal lumen as an isotonic solution in water. It is this fluid and electrolyte secretion into the gut which causes the profound diarrhoea of cholera.

It is important to note that the fluid and electrolyte absorptive mechanism (though clearly swamped by the volume of fluid secreted) is relatively unaffected by the presence of the enterotoxin. It was the appreciation of this fact which opened a new chapter in the management of what are now called "secretory diarrhoeas".

It is now established that other infective diarrhoeas are mediated by a similar mechanism. Enterotoxin-producing *E. coli* are responsible for a wide variety of diarrhoeal illnesses. As much as 70%–80% of "travellers' diarrhoea" has been attributed to enterotoxin-producing *E. coli*, although the incidence varies considerably with geographic location. Pathogenic *E. coli* produce at least two toxins: a heat-labile toxin and a heat-stable toxin. The heat-stable toxin is of lower molecular weight and seems to stimulate intestinal cell secretion via a different intracellular nucleotide mediator. Guanylate cyclase is stimulated by the heat-stable toxin, which catalyses the formation of cyclic guanylate monophosphate (cGMP). Although the kinetics of this reaction are different from those described above for cholera toxin, the net effect is water and electrolyte secretion into the gastrointestinal tract. The effect of the heat-labile toxin produced by *E. coli*, like cholera toxin, is mediated via adenyl cyclase and cAMP, but the magnitude of the activation of adenylate cyclase is considerably less with the consequence that diarrhoea and fluid flux so produced are proportionately smaller.

The pathophysiological mechanisms involved in secretory diarrhoeas are not specific for infection. There is evidence to indicate that several organic molecules such as bile acids, prostaglandins, fatty acids and certain hormones cause diarrhoea by induction of intestinal secretion via the mediation of one or other of the cyclic nucleotides.

In addition to *Vibrio cholerae* and *E. coli*, other bacteria which are known to produce an enterotoxin capable of stimulating small bowel secretion include *Shigella, Staphylococcus aureus, Clostridium perfringens, Clostridium difficile, Pseudomonas aeruginosa, Yersinia enterocolitica* and *Klebsiella pneumoniae*.

Therapeutic Principles

The vast majority of infective diarrhoeas seen in routine practice are self-limiting and require *no* specific therapy other than a simple anti-diarrhoeal agent such as kaolin.

However, for the minority of patients in whom there is a more profound illness, accurate diagnosis is essential. For this, nothing can replace the taking of a full and accurate history and a careful physical examination including a sigmoidoscopy (with rectal biopsy if indicated) and a faecal occult blood test as well as measurement of temperature. The stools should be inspected for consistency, volume and the presence of abnormal constituents such as obvious blood or pus. Microscopy of the stool in infective diarrhoeas is helpful, the presence of pus cells indicating mucosal damage and presumably, therefore, mucosal invasion. Stool culture should be routine and include media which make it possible to identify the growth of *Campylobacter* and *Clostridium difficile* as well as the usual non-lactose fermenting organisms.

In severely ill patients, and particularly in the presence of fever, blood cultures are clearly indicated. Serum should also be obtained at the start of the illness so that retrospective diagnosis will then be made possible from the diagnostic changes of serological titres in convalescent serum.

Persistent secretory diarrhoeas are usually easy to identify as such by observing the 24-h stool volume on a normal diet and comparing this with the 24-h stool volume during fasting. Diarrhoea which is food dependent is likely to be due to secondary phenomena, for example, lactose intolerance, which is particularly common in the days or weeks following infantile enteritis. In secretory diarrhoea the measured osmolality of the stool water should be equal, or virtually so, to that calculated from the measured concentration of the major stool cations (that is, sodium concentration plus potassium concentration multiplied by 2 to account for the anions). An unexplained "osmotic gap" between observed and calculated osmolality frequently indicates the presence of other osmotically active solutes such as unabsorbed carbohydrate or the surreptitious use of laxatives.

The aims of treatment in infective diarrhoea are (a) to relieve the distressing symptoms, (b) to eradicate the infecting organism, (c) to prevent complications and (d) if relevant, to locate the sources of infection and prevent spread.

Management

In practice, therapy in infective diarrhoeas usually begins before an accurate laboratory-based microbiological diagnosis is available. Many patients do not present for medical treatment since their illness is short lived and self-limiting. In those patients who do present, the therapeutic approach is dictated by the clinical assessment of the problem since the severity of the symptoms is so variable.

Generally antibiotic treatment is to be *avoided* (see below), and simple symptomatic treatment should be tried first. But "toxic" patients usually require the diagnostic and therapeutic facilities available to hospital in-patients.

The following are usually successful for symptomatic treatment:

Kaolin compound powder or kaolin mixture 10–20 ml 4 hourly

Codeine phosphate 60–120 mg daily in divided doses. This is an opiate and can cause significant respiratory depression, particularly in children.

Diphenoxylate (usually in the form of Lomotil, which contains a trivial dose of atropine) 10–20 mg daily in divided doses. This is also related to the opiates and can cause similar CNS effects to codeine.

Loperamide 4–16 mg daily in divided doses. This drug is also related to the opiates but is said to be without the CNS effects of codeine and diphenoxolate.

The use of antimicrobial drugs to eradicate the infecting organism is unnecessary in the vast majority of infective diarrhoeas. This is especially so in childhood, where the majority are viral in origin. The patients will usually have cleared the organism spontaneously in 1–3 days but this may be prolonged to a week or more in a few cases. In a small number of cases the patients may retain the organism for a year or more as asymptomatic carriers. The incidence of asymptomatic carriage is greater in the presence of other inflammatory bowel disease. It is now well established that antimicrobial treatment should not be used for infection *limited to the gastrointestinal tract* since this may result in a prolonged period of excretion of the organism and an increase in the eventual number of asymptomatic carriers. Furthermore, there is no clearly demonstrated advantage to be gained from their use in the majority of cases of infective diarrhoea.

However, it is generally agreed that *specific* indications for antimicrobial treatment do exist and these may be summarised as follows:

Typhoid and paratyphoid fever
Cholera
Amoebiasis
Systemic salmonellosis
Yersinia enterocolitica
Giardia lamblia
Severe and prolonged shigellosis
Severe and prolonged *Campylobacter* enteritis

Typhoid and Paratyphoid fever

The clinical picture of enteric fever is produced by infection with *Salmonella typhi* or *Salmonella paratyphi*. The vast majority of the many other *Salmonella* species produce an illness of the "food poisoning" variety in which infecting organisms remain confined to the gastrointestinal tract. However, a few species, such as *Salmonella virchow* and *Salmonella cholerae-suis*, can invade to produce a septicaemic illness similar to enteric fever.

The incubation period for typhoid varies from 1 to 3 weeks but is a little shorter in paratyphoid. The onset is insidious, with fever, headache, cough, constipation and abdominal discomfort which antedate the onset of diarrhoea by about 1 week. The characteristic rash of rose pink macules tends to occur in the 2nd week of the illness. At about this time the rising step-like fever becomes sustained, the abdomen distended and the spleen palpable. The major complications of intestinal perforation or massive haemorrhage tend to occur in the 3rd week of the illness.

Definitive diagnosis is achieved by isolation of the organism from cultures of the blood (maximal yield in the 1st week of the illness) or faeces (maximum positives in the 2nd and 3rd weeks of the illness) and urine (occasionally). Serological diagnosis may be helpful in some cases, but the usefulness of the Widal reaction has been overemphasised in the past.

Treatment

Chloramphenicol probably remains the drug of first choice in enteric fever, given as a 2-week course with a starting dose of 500 mg 4 hourly, decreasing to 500 mg 6 hourly as the fever subsides. In uncomplicated cases response may be expected within 2–4 days. Initially intravenous administration may be indicated when paralytic ileus causes vomiting or when diarrhoea is profound.

Sporadic cases of chloramphenicol-resistant *Salmonella typhi* have been reported and this has become a significant problem in some geographic regions such as South-east Asia and Mexico.

Co-trimoxazole is at least as effective as chloramphenicol in enteric fever and, in the opinion of some, superior to it. It is used orally for 2 weeks in a dose of trimethoprim 160 mg plus sulphamethoxazole 800 mg twice daily. The success of co-trimoxazole is perhaps surprising since *Salmonella typhi* is resistant to sulphonamides alone.

Amoxycillin has proved useful but ampicillin is disappointing.

The treatment of asymptomatic carriers presents a special problem and is, in fact, justifiable only on the grounds of the public's health. Cholecystectomy will eradicate the organism in about two-thirds of carriers but has a surprising morbidity. Co-trimoxazole or amoxycillin are the drugs of choice given for a 4-week course but relapse can occur within 1 or 2 years.

Cholera

A minimum infecting dose of approximately 10^6 *Vibrio cholerae* seems to be necessary in order to produce a clinical illness in normal man. Patients with achlorhydria, however, seem to be more at risk.

Once fluid secretion by the small intestinal mucosa has begun, it seems to be maximal within 4 h and remains so for 4–5 days. Most patients present within 12 h, during which time severe dehydration has often occurred. The clinical picture is therefore that of an apathetic patient with a tachycardia and hypotension and signs of severe fluid depletion in the skin, eyes and mouth. Loss of bicarbonate in the stool results in a metabolic acidosis causing deep sighing respirations and also muscular cramps. Hypokalaemia may be profound.

Treatment

Cholera causes a secretory diarrhoea and systemic invasion by *Vibrio cholerae* is not a problem. The sheet anchor of treatment for cholera, therefore, is the correction and prevention of dehydration by rapid and efficient replacement of fluid and electrolytes. The principles of management are discussed below (page 64). However, it is generally agreed that antibiotic treatment is indicated in cholera for two reasons. Firstly, because antibiotics have been shown to decrease the volume of fluid lost as diarrhoea by as much as 60%. This effect is not noticeable until at least 12 h after administration of the antibiotic (usually tetracycline) but is dramatic by 24–48 h. Secondly, antibiotic treatment shortens the period of excretion of the vibrios in the stool, thus decreasing the period of infectivity.

Tetracycline remains the drug of first choice in cholera, administered orally in a dose of 4 g daily. Co-trimoxazole is probably now the drug of second choice rather than chloramphenicol.

Carrier states occur in approximately 3% of treated patients and can be detected by stool culture following an osmotic purge.

Amoebiasis

This is discussed in detail in Chap. 10. Metronidazole is now the drug of first choice. In amoebic colitis a dose of 400 mg 4 hourly, reducing to 400 mg 6 hourly after 24 h and continuing for 5 days, is advised. In amoebic hepatitis 400 mg 6 hourly is effective. Treatment failures do occur, in which case the second line drugs (chloroquine, emetine hydrochloride) can be used.

Longer courses of treatment may be necessary for the eradication of cysts in asymptomatic carriers.

Systemic Salmonellosis

This is predominantly but not exclusively a disease of childhood in which *Salmonella* infection has not been contained within the gastrointestinal tract, but invasion has occurred, resulting in septicaemic illness in addition to diarrhoea.

Antibiotic resistance develops rapidly in *Salmonella* species. This, combined with previous uncritical antibiotic usage, has resulted in widespread antibiotic resistance among *Salmonella* species. It is therefore essential to culture the infecting organism from blood or faeces in order to examine its antibiotic sensitivities. No single antibiotic is likely to be effective against all *Salmonella* species. If the clinical situation demands treatment before antibiotic sensitivity tests are available, then co-trimoxazole is the drug of first choice.

Yersinia enterocolitica

This organism has long been recognised as pathogenic in Europe and more recently in North America but there seem to be quite marked regional variations in its occurrence. *Yersinia* tends to invade the distal small intestine, producing an illness which may mimic acute appendicitis or Crohn's disease.

Yersinia pseudotuberculosis can produce an acute mesenteric adenitis.

Most illnesses caused by this organism are self-limiting, but outbreaks of severe septicaemic illness are well-recognised and have a significant mortality when diagnosis is delayed. Human-to-human spread almost certainly occurs but domestic animals seem to be the major source in sporadic cases. Diagnosis is by culture of the organism, a slow-growing gram-negative rod, but serology is also frequently used. The organism has a wide range of antibiotic sensitivities. Resistance to several antibiotics, including ampicillin, carbenicillin and chloramphenicol, is well described. Co-trimoxazole is again the drug of first choice, but good results have been achieved with many others, including sulphonamides, aminoglycosides and tetracyclines.

Giardia lamblia

This is a common protozoon parasite. *Local* mucosal invasion has been described, but this is trivial and apparently of no significance. The symptoms of diarrhoea are secondary to malabsorption, which occurs because of the sheer number of parasites adherent to the small intestinal mucosa. These features of steatorrhoea (frequent pale, bulky and offensive motions with abdominal distension, colic, nausea and weight loss) enable giardiasis to be distinguished from other infective diarrhoeas with relative ease. Definitive diagnosis is achieved by finding the cystic forms on stool microscopy, but a higher diagnostic yield results from inspection of jejunal aspirates or biopsies for the trophozoite.

Metronidazole 400 mg three times daily by mouth is highly effective but may need to be continued for up to 10 days.

Giardiasis commonly coexists with other small intestinal disease such as tropical sprue or common variable immune deficiency.

Shigella Dysentery

The four *Shigella* species produce a clinically similar illness but of varying severity. Unlike *Salmonella* or *Vibrio cholerae*, a minute infecting dose can produce a clinical illness. Spread is by the faeco-oral route and organisms multiply rapidly in the colon, where invasion occurs. The clinical features of fever, abdominal pain and diarrhoea are, of course, non-specific, but the onset of bloody diarrhoea and the intense, burning peri-anal pain on defaecation are highly suggestive. The symptoms of inflammatory disease of the rectum are usually marked; that is, very frequent but small amounts of liquid stool with tenesmus and incontinence.

Diagnosis is achieved by isolation of the organism from the stool. Rectal swabs give the lowest yield of positive cultures and the mucous portions of liquid stools give the highest yield. Although systemic symptoms such as meningism and pleuritic chest pain are well described, it is unusual to obtain the organism from blood culture.

The illness is of varying severity and can be mild, particularly when caused by *Shigella sonnei*. For this reason, and also because antibiotic resistance is a frequent and increasing problem, specific antimicrobial treatment is reserved for the severe or prolonged attack. As is the case with all invasive organisms, the antibiotic used should be absorbable and the choice is based on the observed sensitivities of the isolate. If treatment needs to be started before the results are available, then the drugs of first choice are: co-trimoxazole as trimethoprim 80 mg plus sulphamethoxazole 400 mg daily for 5 days or ampicillin 2 g daily for 5 days.

Chronic carriers of *Shigella* have been treated by purgation with lactulose but the relapse rate is unacceptable. However, co-trimoxazole is an effective alternative. As in severe inflammatory bowel disease, such as acute exacerbations of ulcerative colitis, anti-diarrhoeal agents of the opiate group and their analogues are *contra-indicated*. There is evidence to indicate that these drugs can precipitate the development of toxic dilation of the colon.

Campylobacter enteritis

Campylobacter species have been well recognised as an enteric pathogen in veterinary practice for many years, but have only recently emerged as a significant pathogen in humans in the past 10 years. This is not due to any epidemiological change but simply a recognition of the organism's significance in human disease. Now that the organism's fastidious requirements for culture are routinely catered for, it has emerged as quite a common cause of bacterial diarrhoea in man, perhaps accounting for as many as 7% of cases.

A typical attack occurs after an incubation period of usually less than 1 week with a prodrome of malaise, headache, abdominal pain and fever. Diarrhoea then occurs as the abdominal pain becomes colicky. The liquid stool may be accompanied by fresh blood with the result that the illness is sometimes misdiagnosed as ulcerative colitis—an error which may be compounded by the superficial resemblance of the diseased rectal mucosa to the sigmoidoscopic appearance of ulcerative colitis.

Diagnosis is achieved by isolation of the organism from a pus-containing stool. Phase-contrast microscopy of *fresh* stool will also enable the *Campylobacter* species to be recognised by their characteristic darting and oscillating movements.

It is difficult to assess the overall incidence of antibiotic resistance. The organism's fastidious cultural requirements make sensitivity studies difficult and no good clinical trials are available. It is generally agreed, however, that erythromycin, tetracycline, the aminoglycosides (especially gentamycin) and nitrofurans are highly effective whereas the penicillin group, co-trimoxazole, cephalosporins and lincomycin are ineffective.

Because erythromycin is narrow in spectrum, safe and effective, it is regarded as the drug of first choice in a dose of 500 mg twice daily. Many cases resolve spontaneously before the organism is isolated.

Management of Fluid and Electrolyte Depletion

Many more patients, especially in the very old and very young age groups, die from thromboembolism and other complications of dehydration than from bacterial invasion. Thus the overriding priority in all forms of diarrhoea is the correction of dehydration and the associated electrolyte depletion. In extreme cases rehydration is carried out with sterile isotonic electrolyte solutions intravenously. But the lessons of cholera are now being more widely applied in other diarrhoeal diseases.

In the torrential diarrhoea of cholera the large volumes of sterile intravenous fluids are prohibitively expensive in those areas of the third world where cholera is prevalent. However, as discussed previously, the diarrhoea of cholera results from the secretion of water and electrolytes by the gastrointestinal mucosa. The absorptive process is relatively unaffected. Consequently, if glucose is placed in the intestinal lumen it is absorbed normally by an active transport process. The absorption of glucose is coupled with sodium absorption so that both are absorbed concurrently. The absorption of sodium and glucose results in the absorption of water by solvent drag. Thus, in cholera and indeed in any secretory diarrhoea, the fluid and electrolyte loss may be treated by the administration of large volumes of glucose-electrolyte solutions by mouth. The composition of the glucose electrolyte solutions used in early work was based on the electrolyte concentrations of the water from choleraic stools. These solutions have been refined so that at present the optimum mixture for cholera is as follows:

Glucose 110 mEq/litre
Sodium 99 mEq/litre
Chloride 74 mEq/litre
Bicarbonate 39 mEq/litre
Potassium 14 mEq/litre

Similar solutions can be used for secretory diarrhoeas other than cholera. The optimum concentrations of electrolytes and precisely which "carrier molecule" is preferable in various clinical situations continues to be debated. But at present no solution seems to have significant advantages over the World Health Organisation glucose solution for non-cholera diarrhoea, the composition of which is:

Glucose 20 g/litre
Sodium 90 mEq/litre
Chloride 75 mEq/litre
Bicarbonate 30 mEq/litre
Potassium 15 mEq/litre

These solutions do not decrease the diarrhoea but allow hydration to be maintained simply, safely and cheaply. They are now in common usage in the enteritis of infancy and in those infective diarrhoeas of adults which are particularly severe or prolonged. However, as knowledge of the biochemical mechanisms involved in secretory diarrhoeas improves, hopes of a pharmacological approach to the control of diarrhoea are beginning to emerge and various pharmacological agents have been recommended to decrease the fluid output in secretory diarrhoea. Some of these agents interfere with the production or elimination of cyclic nucleotides. In the laboratory this can be achieved (a) by blocking the receptor to prevent enterotoxin binding to epithelial cell membranes (for example with fragments of cholera enterotoxin molecule), (b) by preventing the stimulation of adenyl or guanylate cyclase (for example with propranolol, chlorpromazine or adenosine analogues) or (c) by increasing the rate of removal of the cyclic nucleotide.

This pharmacological approach is as yet in its infancy, and the mechanism of action of many agents remains unknown. Prostaglandin synthetase inhibitors such as indomethacin or salicylates will undoubtedly decrease the fluid output by the small intestinal mucosa in the experimental situation, but their site of action is unknown. Similarly, ethacrynic acid and corticosteroid will reverse the intestinal secretion induced by cholera toxin by an unknown mechanism. Some of these agents, such as chlorpromazine and (sometimes) corticosteroids, can produce useful therapeutic results in clinical practice although their true role in management has yet to be determined. Others, such as propranolol and indomethacin, have not in the clinical situation fulfilled their promise as suggested by their effects in the laboratory.

Further Reading

Field M, Fordtran JS, Schultz SG (1980) Secretory diarrhoea. Clinical physiology series. American Physiological Society, Bethesda
Lambert HP (ed) (1979) Infections of the G.I. tract. Clin. Gastroenterol 8(3) Saunders, London Philadelphia Toronto

5 Inflammatory Bowel Disease
B. T. Cooper

Introduction

Inflammatory bowel disease (IBD) is an all-embracing term for the idiopathic chronic inflammatory disorders of the intestine, ulcerative colitis and Crohn's disease (regional enteritis). In the U.S.A. there is a tendency to restrict its usage to ulcerative and Crohn's colitis. In this chapter, the first section will discuss the various treatments which have been claimed to suppress inflammation, induce or maintain remissions and alter the course of IBD; their place in current management is assessed. The second part of the chapter considers the management of ulcerative colitis, Crohn's colitis, Crohn's disease of the small intestine, the complications of IBD and IBD in the special situations of pregnancy, old age and childhood.

Perhaps in the foreseeable future, the cause of IBD will be known and a curative therapy may then be available. Until then, we have to acknowledge that there is no pharmacological cure for IBD. Nevertheless, the management of IBD is undergoing continual change and evolution as new ideas and therapies are introduced and submitted to assessment. The disease is most effectively managed by physicians and surgeons working together. Many aspects of the management of IBD are still controversial, and perhaps none more so than the roles of azathioprine and surgery in the management of Crohn's disease.

Treatments Used in Inflammatory Bowel Disease

Drugs

Corticosteroids

Corticosteroids are used to suppress inflammation in IBD. This action is non-specific and individuals vary considerably in their response. All studies, however, have shown corticosteroids to be of benefit in the treatment of IBD, and they form the basis of drug therapy in many cases. However, it is important to emphasise that a diagnosis of IBD does not automatically mean that the patient requires steroid therapy. The main indications are acute severe or moderately severe active disease and chronic persistent active disease. Corticosteroids are also indicated for some of the complications of IBD (see p 84). There is no evidence that they are of any value in maintenance of remissions, prevention of relapses or altering the course of the disease whether it be ulcerative colitis, Crohn's colitis or Crohn's disease of the small intestine. Indeed, there is some evidence that the recurrence rate is increased in patients with Crohn's disease on corticosteroids. This appears to be only partly explained by the fact that they are given in more severe or extensive cases. Deaths may be more common in the corticosteroid-treated patients with Crohn's disease and are not only related to the severity of Crohn's disease in these patients but also to the complications of such treatment.

The most widely used corticosteroid is prednisolone by mouth and, of course, it can be associated with any of the steroid side-effects, particularly when more than 7.5 mg per day is given. Side-effects may be reduced by an alternative day steroid regime. Indigestion is one of the commonest problems, even with small doses, and may be alleviated by the use of enteric-coated tablets. Some physicians prefer ACTH because it may have fewer side-effects overall and because it seems easier to wean patients off it. However, ACTH may be more prone to cause acne and hypertension than prednisolone. During severe attacks or at the time of surgery, hydrocortisone sodium succinate or prednisolone sodium phosphate may be given intravenously. A danger of corticosteroids is that they may mask the symptoms of free perforation of the bowel. In patients with proctitis, distal colitis or extensive colitis with troublesome rectal symptoms (i.e. urgency, bleeding and tenesmus), retention enemas of prednisolone disodium phosphate or hydrocortisone acetate may be useful in suppressing inflammation locally. Enema fluid has been shown to pass around the colon as far as the midtransverse colon. There is evidence that up to 40% of steroid administered rectally may be absorbed, so adrenal suppression may be a problem. However, while patients on steroid enemata long term have evidence of slight adrenal suppression, there are no reports of it being clinically important. Hydrocortisone acetate foam enemata are available, and although the foam does not pass beyond the splenic flexure, it does seem to be as effective clinically as fluid retention enemata. Retention of enemata may be difficult or impossible for elderly patients and for those with severe tenesmus. In these patients, the foam may be retained more easily.

Sulphasalazine

Sulphasalazine is made up of sulphapyridine and 5-aminosalicylic acid linked by an azo bond. It is used in two situations in IBD: as maintenance therapy and as a suppressor of inflammatory activity. There is good evidence that sulphasalazine maintains remissions and reduces the risk of relapse in ulcerative colitis. This appears to be dose related. However, the weight of the evidence suggests that it is of no value as maintenance therapy in Crohn's disease of the colon or small intestine. There is no evidence that maintenance sulphasalazine alters the course of either form of IBD. There is little objective evidence that sulphasalazine is of value in suppressing active inflammation in ulcerative colitis. However, most physicians will have seen patients with mild or moderate ulcerative colitis who seem to respond to it. There is some preliminary evidence from the U.S.A. that sulphasalazine may suppress inflammatory activity in Crohn's colitis and possibly even in small intestinal Crohn's disease, although most physicians have yet to be convinced. Sulphasalazine, therefore, should certainly be tried in patients with mild to moderate colitis before resorting to steroids.

The mechanism of action of sulphasalazine is unknown, although it may suppress prostaglandin synthetase activity, which has been shown to increase in the colonic mucosa during flare-ups of ulcerative colitis. The drug is partly absorbed whole in the small intestine and the remaining unabsorbed drug is broken down by colonic bacteria to sulphapyridine and 5-aminosalicylic acid, which are excreted in the faeces. There is now good evidence that the latter component is the "active ingredient". Both sulphasalazine and 5-aminosalicylic acid enemata have been used with benefit in proctitis whereas sulphapyridine enemata are useless. 5-Aminosalicylic acid has not been given by mouth but it would be absorbed in the small intestine and, therefore, may be of little value as its main effect seems to be local in the colon. Side-effects of sulphasalazine are common (1%–5%) and include skin rashes, fever, nausea, lethargy and depression, marrow depression, haemolysis, macrocytosis with or without folate deficiency, apparently reversible azoospermia and hepatotoxicity. Indigestion is common and may improve with enteric-coated tablets. Some if not all of the side-effects are commoner in slow acetylators of the drug and are associated with high serum levels of sulphapyridine.

Disodium Cromoglycate (DSCG)

Disodium cromoglycate is an expensive drug which has been promoted as a therapy for ulcerative colitis because it was thought that type I hypersensitivity reactions might be involved in exacerbations of the disease. However, a majority of the controlled trials show that oral DSCG (as Nalcrom) has no advantage over placebo in suppressing acute attacks and is not as good as sulphasalazine in maintaining remissions. However, the occasional patient with ulcerative colitis does seem to benefit from oral DSCG but, of course, a placebo response cannot be excluded. DSCG enemata, however, may benefit patients with idiopathic proctitis who have large numbers of eosinophils and IgE-containing plasma cells in their rectal mucosa. These patients have been classified as having allergic proctitis. DSCG does not prevent relapses in Crohn's disease.

Immunosuppressants

Azathioprine

Azathioprine is a purine antagonist which destroys immunologically competent cells. It is metabolised in the body to 6-mercaptopurine. It has been used in both ulcerative colitis and Crohn's disease. In ulcerative colitis there is little evidence that azathioprine confers any advantage over steroids on their own in the suppression of inflammatory activity. In patients with chronic ulcerative colitis who are on continuous steroids, addition of azathioprine allows reduction of the steroid dose without a change in symptoms.

In spite of initial enthusiasm, there is little evidence that azathioprine is of value in the suppression of inflammation in Crohn's disease. As in ulcerative colitis, azathioprine allows a reduction in steroid dosage without relapse of symptoms in patients with chronic disease. Most studies suggest that azathioprine is of no value in maintaining a remission induced by medical or surgical therapy and does not alter the long-term course of Crohn's disease. There is no real place for azathioprine in the treatment of IBD except for its possible value as a steroid-sparing agent. However, it must be said that the occasional severely ill patient with Crohn's disease may remit when steroids alone have failed. Also there is anecdotal evidence that azathioprine may heal enterocutaneous fistulae in Crohn's disease, although evidence is lacking from controlled trials.

6-Mercaptopurine (6-MP)

This metabolite of azathioprine has been extensively used in IBD by one group from New York. Their results appear impressive until one realises that their ulcerative colitis and some of their Crohn's disease studies are uncontrolled. In their controlled studies, 6-MP does seem to be of value in reducing relapses and maintaining remission in patients with Crohn's colitis and with small intestinal disease. 6-MP has not been studied elsewhere, so one must be cautious in regarding it as an advance in the treatment of Crohn's disease. Moreover it is difficult to reconcile the apparent benefit of 6-MP with the lack of benefit of its precursor, azathioprine.

Common side-effects of azathioprine and 6-MP are nausea, fever and sepsis, but marrow suppression is by far the most important one and as a result these drugs can rarely be justified in the treatment of IBD. Moreover, the potential long-term risk of defective immune surveillance as well as the risk of sterility, mutagenicity and teratogenicity should make the physician very wary of their use in diseases which commonly affect young people.

Thalidomide

Thalidomide suppresses lepra reactions, possibly by an effect on immune complexes. There is anecdotal evidence of its benefit in chronic ulcerative colitis; however, in view of its teratogenicity its use is not recommended.

Levamisole

This immunostimulant drug enhances impaired phagocyte and T-lymphocyte function. An initial uncontrolled study suggested that levamisole was of benefit in maintaining remissions in patients with Crohn's disease, but controlled trials have failed to confirm this. The main side-effects are granulocytopenia, rashes and drug-induced arthritis and its use is not recommended in Crohn's disease.

Antimicrobials

Broad Spectrum Antibiotics

Although quite extensively used in the past, there is no evidence to suggest that broad spectrum antibiotics are of any value in the treatment of IBD. Indeed, they often appear to produce a relapse of ulcerative colitis or Crohn's colitis. Antibiotics are only indicated in a few defined situations such as abscess, infection and probably toxic megacolon and peri-operatively to prevent surgical sepsis.

Metronidazole

Controlled trials with metronidazole have failed to show that it is of any benefit in patients with either ulcerative colitis or Crohn's disease. However, patients with peri-anal Crohn's disease and sepsis may have considerable symptomatic improvement with metronidazole, presumably related to its effect on anaerobic organisms. Side-effects include rashes, dizziness, headache and a weak disulfiram-like interaction with alcohol.

Non-drug Therapies

Zinc Replacement

Plasma zinc levels, which poorly reflect total body stores of zinc, are normal in ulcerative colitis but may vary with disease activity in Crohn's disease. Oral zinc supplements have no therapeutic benefit in ulcerative colitis. Patients with small intestinal Crohn's disease can very occasionally develop zinc deficiency with symptoms which are correctable by zinc replacement. However, there is, as yet, no evidence that zinc deficiency or its treatment is important in Crohn's disease.

BCG

General immune stimulation with recurrent oral doses of BCG has not proved beneficial in patients with Crohn's disease.

Plasmapheresis

Plasmapheresis may remove antibodies and immune complexes from the patient's blood and has been used in one preliminary uncontrolled trial in chronic Crohn's disease. The patients seemed able to decrease steroid dosage without relapse during plasmaphoresis and some relapses seemed to settle on plasmapheresis alone. However, it is possible that these were spontaneous remissions given the relapsing and remitting nature of the disease.

Transfer Factor

The transfer of immunologically active substances from healthy blood to patients with Crohn's disease was suggested to be beneficial in one uncontrolled study, but in the only controlled study so far performed it had no advantage over placebo.

Nutritional Support

Hyperalimentation with total parenteral nutrition (TPN), elemental diet or enteral nutrition has been used in patients with Crohn's disease. While there are some reports of dramatic remissions during hyperalimentation, overall one has to conclude that convincing evidence for its therapeutic benefit is lacking. There are also reports of the healing of chronic enterocutaneous fistulae with bowel rest and TPN or elemental diet. The main role for nutritional support appears to be in patients with extensive small intestinal resection, in patients in a poor nutritional state (especially with extensive active disease or if surgery is being considered) and in children with growth failure secondary to Crohn's disease. When possible, enteral nutrition usually via a fine polyethylene nasogastric feeding tube is to be preferred to the more expensive and potentially hazardous TPN. However, with extensive small bowel resection, a period of TPN may be inevitable. TPN may be indicated for bowel rest in an attempt to heal a fistula. For patients who can be fed by mouth, there is no real evidence that elemental diets have any advantage over enteral nutrition, which is usually cheaper and is well tolerated.

There is no evidence that nutritional support is valuable in the treatment of ulcerative colitis per se, although it may be indicated in patients with acute colitis peri-operatively and in poorly nourished patients with active disease.

Diet

Patients are usually advised to eat a high protein, high calorie diet with no further specific instructions. Special diets that are occasionally required are lactose-free for patients with coexistent lactase deficiency, low roughage for patients with small intestinal Crohn's disease and a tendency to obstruction, high roughage for patients with IBD who are also constipated or have colon spasm and low fat for patients with small intestinal Crohn's disease with steatorrhoea. Until recently no one seriously thought that diet might have a therapeutic role in the management of IBD. However, there have been a number of studies which, although open to severe criticism of their methodology, suggest that patients with Crohn's disease eat more refined carbohydrate before the onset of their disease than controls or patients with ulcerative colitis. Whether this observation is of value therapeutically is not known, but one retrospective study has suggested that patients taking a low refined carbohydrate diet had fewer resections and admissions to hospital than patients from a control group on undefined diets, looked after by different physicians and often in different hospitals. Many are sceptical as to whether dietary manipulation offers an exciting therapeutic breakthrough in the treatment of Crohn's disease, but prospective controlled trials are now taking place to answer this question.

Psychotherapy

There is no evidence that formal psychotherapy is of benefit in treating flare-ups or maintaining remissions in IBD. However, patients often describe relapses following emotional upset, and most physicians hold the view that patients seem to do better if they are closely followed up in a special clinic run by interested, concerned, approachable and experienced gastroenterologists. There is no incontrovertible evidence for this, but it would help to explain the frequency with which new drugs or treatments seem to work in uncontrolled situations.

Management of Ulcerative Colitis and Crohn's Colitis

Ulcerative colitis is a chronic relapsing mucosal inflammatory disorder of unknown aetiology; it is cured by panproctocolectomy. Crohn's colitis is a chronic relapsing mucosal and submucosal granulomatous inflammatory disorder of unknown aetiology which is symptomatically similar to ulcerative colitis. Although Crohn's colitis may be differentiated from ulcerative colitis by mucosal appearance, histology, radiological appearances, patchiness of the lesions, rectal sparing, association with peri-anal disease (tags, fissures, fistulae) in practice this is often difficult. Crohn's colitis tends to be more troublesome than ulcerative colitis in that it relapses more often and more seriously and is more likely to lead to definitive surgery. However, colectomy does not cure the disorder because of the possibility of recurrent disease in the small intestine. While it is of some value prognostically to differentiate between the two disorders, in practice, management of both disorders is largely the same. Indeed, there is a tendency, particularly in the U.S.A., to make no real attempt to separate one from the other. This approach has some merit, especially as many cases are very difficult to separate and not infrequently typical cases of ulcerative colitis are found to have a colon full of granulomata after colectomy.

In this discussion of the treatment, the two disorders will be considered together and any differences will be highlighted as necessary.

Aims of Treatment

The aims of treatment of colitis are to keep the patient symptom free, to suppress inflammatory activity should it prove a problem, to avoid relapses and to screen for and treat complications as and when they arise. As there is no definitive medical therapy, treatment is directed towards explanation, reassurance of the patient and relatives and provision of support and advice where needed. It is important to make the patients feel that their disease is continually being thought about and that therapy is rational and planned, not haphazard and responding to events.

Follow Up

It is important to remember that either type of colitis is a chronic disorder and that patients need lifelong follow up. Even after colectomy and ileostomy, follow up is required because of the risk of mechanical problems with the stoma, metabolic problems, prestomal ileitis and, in Crohn's colitis, recurrent disease.

Most gastroenterological physicians would agree that follow up should be in a special clinic where the physicians have experience in managing IBD and where the patient will be seen as often as necessary by the same physician, with whom a good relationship can be built up. It is important that patients have easy access to the clinic. Management should be largely in the hands of physicians but a gastroenterological surgical opinion should be easily available. This is often best achieved by a combined medical–surgical clinic. Dieticians, stoma therapists and nurses with experience in managing the problems of IBD patients should be present in the clinic.

Diagnosis and Assessment

To make the diagnosis and to provide baseline information against which the progress of the disease can be assessed, the following are necessary after a full history and examination, including sigmoidoscopy: visual stool inspection, stool microscopy and culture, rectal biopsy (provided the colitis is not very severe), full blood count, differential white cell count, erythrocyte sedimentation rate (ESR) (or acute phase protein, e.g. orosomucoid, C reactive protein), blood urea, electrolytes, calcium and magnesium, serum proteins, liver function tests, iron and total iron binding capacity (or transferrin), and plain X-ray of the abdomen (in severe acute colitis) or barium enema (provided the colitis is not severe). Further tests may be warranted in certain situations: barium follow-through (or small bowel enema) if associated small intestinal disease is suspected, colonoscopy with biopsy if diagnosis is difficult or if dysplasia or carcinoma is suspected, tests of malabsorption if associated small intestinal disease is present, serum folate if the patient is taking sulphasalazine and tests of coagulation if a coexisting or complicating bleeding diathesis is suspected. In follow up it is important to examine the patient and to repeat sigmoidoscopy with biopsy at appropriate intervals. The following blood tests are mandatory as abnormalities of them may indicate continued inflammatory activity: haemoglobin, white cell count, ESR and serum albumin; repeat barium studies and/or colonoscopy are necessary to assess the extent of the disease. Other tests may need to be repeated as indicated.

Severe Colitis

Patients with colitis who have severe bloody diarrhoea with nausea, vomiting, abdominal distension and tenderness with or without rebound tenderness, who are febrile, look ill, are dehydrated and have a tachycardia, and who have evidence of active disease as shown by a low haemoglobin, low serum albumin, a neutrophil leucocytosis and a raised ESR may be considered to have severe colitis. These may be features of an acute presentation of the disease or of an acute relapse. These patients should be admitted without delay for bedrest. After examination a gentle sigmoidoscopy using minimal air should be performed. In acute colitis rectal instrumentation can help to precipitate toxic megacolon. Similarly, rectal biopsy and barium enema should be avoided until the patient is better. However, a plain abdominal X-ray is mandatory to assess the degree of colonic dilatation and to seek evidence of perforation, and often a good picture of colonic mucosa and the extent of the inflammation can be gained by the air contrast appearance of gas in the colon.

The patient should have an intravenous catheter inserted and electrolyte and fluid losses should be replaced with special consideration of potassium, for hypokalaemia may precipitate toxic megacolon. Patients are frequently anaemic and blood transfusion should keep their haemoglobin normal. If the patient is vomiting, a nasogastric tube should be passed. Initially the patient should take nothing by mouth except sips of water. High dose parenteral steroids should be started at once in the form of prednisolone sodium phosphate 60–80 mg/day or the equivalent dose of hydrocortisone sodium succinate. In very severe fulminating cases when toxic megacolon is thought to be a real possibility, it is probably wise to start parenteral broad spectrum antibiotics which include cover for faecal anaerobes. Sulphasalazine, azathioprine and anticholinergics have no place in the therapy of acute severe colitis. Anti-diarrhoeal agents are contra-indicated as they may precipitate toxic megacolon. Opiate analgesics have the same risk so pain relief can be a major problem in severe colitis and there is no satisfactory answer. If analgesia is really necessary, initially paracetamol orally may be tried but if this does not work, careful use of buprenorphine may be indicated. Aspirin and other non-steroid anti-inflammatory analgesics are not indicated.

After admission, the gastroenterological surgical team should be notified, for management is jointly medical and surgical. A plan of care should be formulated at the outset, whereby medical treatment is allowed to proceed for a certain period and if at the end of this time there is not a *definite* improvement, surgery should proceed. The period of medical treatment is determined by many factors, including the patient's age, severity of colitis, previous health and nutrition. However, usually the period allowed for improvement on medical treatment is 24–48 h. Obviously, rapid deterioration or a sudden complication such as colonic perforation or profound haemorrhage may precipitate earlier surgery. Toxic dilatation is considered by some as an indication for surgery in itself, but others would give patients up to 24 h to improve before proceeding to surgery. It is always tempting to delay surgery in the hope that the patient will improve, but this is what often leads to disaster since deterioration may be very sudden, the patient's general condition will be much worse and the optimum time for surgery will have passed. It is better to operate too early than too late and it is better for one panproctocolectomy to be performed in a patient who might have recovered if left than for a patient to die because surgery was delayed. Admittedly deadlines for surgery may need to be slightly more flexible in patients with Crohn's colitis as the decision to operate may be complicated by the presence of coexistent small intestinal disease, but in these patients if there is no definite response to medical therapy, surgery should proceed at once.

Continued medical management consists of continuing intravenous fluids (with special attention paid to potassium replacement), parenteral steroids in high doses and antibiotics, water only by mouth and blood transfusions to keep the haemoglobin normal. This regime should be continued for 5–7 days provided the patient is recovering. Nutrition may be a problem, but if the patient was previously well nourished a few days without calories is not disadvantageous; on the other hand if the patient was previously poorly nourished, TPN should be started at the outset. During the early phase of intense therapy, it is necessary to measure the pulse, temperature and blood pressure 4 hourly, to examine the abdomen and measure its girth daily, to measure haemoglobin, urea and electrolytes daily, to obtain a daily plain X-ray film of the abdomen to assess colonic size and to record accurately stool frequency, appearance and weight.

Improvement is shown by improvement in well-being, fall in temperature and pulse rate, and lessening abdominal pain, abdominal distension and diarrhoea. Biochemical and haematological indices of inflammatory activity may recover slowly. After the intense 5–7 day course the antibiotics are stopped and the steroids are given orally and feeding by mouth instituted. Some patients may relapse at this stage and this is an indication for surgery. Patients do not seem to do well with repeated courses of intensive parenteral therapy. During recovery, diet should be high in proteins and calories. In some patients, especially the elderly, feeding may be difficult and enteral nutrition via a fine nasogastric feeding tube is indicated. It is always worth avoiding TPN in this recovery phase. After the patient has been on oral steroids for about a week, the prednisolone dose can be reduced by 2.5–5.0 mg every 2–4 days and sulphasalazine 1 g three times a day started. In this recovery phase the aim is to help the patient to full recovery with good diet and plenty of bed rest, and too early discharge is unwise. The patient may need oral iron supplements. At the time of discharge the prednisolone dose should be about 20 mg/day. Patients with colitis are at great risk of venous thrombo-embolic disease, so gentle physiotherapy should be started as soon as possible after improvement begins and daily examination should include examination of the legs and chest.

Moderate Colitis

Patients with bloody diarrhoea, perhaps nausea and abdominal discomfort, slight fever, and haematological and biochemical signs of activity may be considered to have moderate colitis. These patients usually need to be admitted although sometimes they can be managed on an out-patient basis, provided they can be seen frequently. After full clinical assessment with sigmoidoscopy and baseline investigations, treatment is usually started with prednisolone (or equivalent) 20–40 mg daily by mouth unless the patient is very nauseated or vomiting. Sulphasalazine, 1 g three times a day, can be started at the same time. It is important to remember that moderate colitis does not always require steroids and some patients will settle with bed rest and sulphasalazine alone. Diet should be high protein and high calorie and oral iron supplements may be necessary. If the haemoglobin level is less than 10 g/100 ml, the patient should be transfused to raise the level to normal. Hypokalaemia can be corrected by oral supplements. If symptoms of rectal involvement such as tenesmus or urgency are a problem, the patient may gain relief from hydrocortisone or prednisolone retention enemata once or twice a day. Some patients may settle with steroid enemata rather than oral steroids. As symptoms improve, oral steroids can be progressively and fairly rapidly cut down to a dose of prednisolone 10–20 mg by the time of discharge. Anti-diarrhoeal agents are not contra-indicated in moderate colitis but may be of limited value in patients with bad colonic inflammation. Their use should be closely monitored. Pain may be helped by anticholinergics but it usually is not severe and requires no specific therapy.

Mild Colitis

Patients with bloody diarrhoea, perhaps mild abdominal discomfort, but no fever and nausea and little haematological or biochemical evidence of activity are considered to have mild colitis and can be treated on an out-patient basis. Some patients may settle with reassurance and anti-diarrhoeals alone. Many require further treatment with sulphasalazine 1 g three times a day and, especially if the colitis is left-sided, steroid retention enemata once or twice per day. A very few patients may require a short sharp course of oral steroids. Anticholinergics may be helpful in those few patients with a lot of colonic pain and spasm.

Therapy Between Exacerbations

The aim of maintenance therapy is to keep the patient as symptom free as possible and to reduce the risk of recurrence. As steroids do not reduce the risk of recurrence, prednisolone should be reduced by 5 mg approximately every 2 weeks to 10 mg provided there is no relapse. Then prednisolone should be slowly decreased until it is stopped. The decrease may have to be as little as 1 mg every week or fortnight to prevent relapse. Patients may have to be actively encouraged to reduce the dose as they miss the sense of well-being that steroids impart, even though there has been no relapse of colitis. If the patient relapses, it is necessary to increase the dose temporarily and start reduction again when the patient is reasonably well. It can, however, prove impossible to stop steroids completely in some patients. Patients with Crohn's colitis are much more likely to require a maintenance dose of steroids to control symptoms than patients with ulcerative colitis. Patients with ulcerative colitis are maintained on sulphasalazine indefinitely as this drug has been shown to reduce the risk of relapse. This benefit has not been shown with Crohn's disease but most patients with Crohn's colitis are maintained on sulphasalazine. Sulphasalazine side-effects are common (1%–5% of patients), and those with fever or drug rash may be desensitised by starting with minute doses, such as 1 mg per day, and building up to the conventional therapeutic dose. In patients with distal disease, symptoms may be controlled with regular steroid enemata and with oral sulphasalazine. Patients can then usefully control their disease by taking steroid retention enemata at night only when they see blood in their stool.

During follow up, some patients, especially young women, may be liable to iron deficiency and this should be treated appropriately. Patients on sulphasalazine may be liable to folate deficiency, which is easily corrected with oral folic acid 5 mg twice daily.

There are usually no obvious causes for relapses of colitis but stress, broad spectrum antibiotics and intercurrent (especially gastrointestinal) infections may be associated with relapse.

If patients with ulcerative colitis have diarrhoea without much evidence of activity of the colitis, lactase deficiency (which occasionally is seen in colitis) should be considered and if present, treated with a lactose-free diet. Similarly, diarrhoea occurring in a patient with seemingly inactive Crohn's colitis may be related to involvement of the small intestine (see p. 79).

Idiopathic Proctitis

Patients with idiopathic proctitis have disease limited to the rectum and lower sigmoid colon. The symptoms are usually bloody diarrhoea with or without left iliac fossa discomfort. Histologically the disease is usually identical to ulcerative colitis, although a few cases will present features of Crohn's colitis. In 30% of these patients, the disease progresses proximally to total or subtotal colitis. In the remainder, the disease remains limited to the distal colon and rectum and prognosis is excellent. Many of these patients have a long history of constipation and they frequently relate the passage of hard stools to rectal bleeding. In this group, the aim of treatment is to eliminate constipation with a high-fibre diet. However, some may require additional therapy with a preparation such as lactulose. With adequate treatment, there is little problem with hard or loose stools or blood. In the majority who are not constipated, treatment consists of steroid retention enemata and sulphasalazine by mouth. They very rarely require oral steroids. Patients with "allergic" proctitis may be helped by DSCG by mouth or enema.

Surgery

The indications for surgery in colitis are:

Absolute indications:
   Acute fulminating colitis
   Carcinoma
   Perforation

Usual indications:
   Massive haemorrhage
   Toxic megacolon

Occasional indications:
   Arthritis
   Growth failure (children)
   Peri-anal disease (rare in ulcerative colitis)
   Persistent disease
   Pyoderma gangrenosum
   Stricture

The complications of colitis are discussed later. Gastrointestinal surgeons should be involved in the treatment of colitis and, whenever possible, therapy should be planned with them. It is a mistake to regard surgery as necessary only when medical therapy has failed or when the patient has earned his operation by tolerating his symptoms for so long. Medical and surgical therapy are complementary and it is always better to plan surgery and perform a total colectomy electively for the mortality is 1%–2% compared with up to 20% for emergency colectomy.

The operation of choice in either type of colitis is panproctocolectomy with ileostomy. In an emergency situation, the operation may have to be performed in two stages with a colectomy and ileostomy at the time and an elective proctectomy at a later date. Most satisfactory results are obtained with the standard Brooke 'spout' ileostomy but in specialised centres the continent ileostomy with a Kock pouch may be possible. However, even in the special centres there is a high incidence of postoperative complications, a high re-operation rate and a significant operative mortality with the continent ileostomy.

Patients with an aversion to an ileostomy can be offered a colectomy with ileorectal anastomosis provided that they have a reasonable rectal capacity and they realise that they will have to accept increased stool frequency, often with urgency, and that the remaining rectum is still at risk from carcinoma and can still cause symptoms of bloody diarrhoea and tenesmus which may require local or systemic therapy. Many patients eventually have to have a proctectomy and ileostomy. Ileorectal anastomosis is contra-indicated in the emergency situation and if peri-anal disease is present. However, this operation can give good results with Crohn's colitis with rectal sparing.

Crohn's colitis has occasionally been treated in certain centres by a diversionary ileostomy without colectomy. It is claimed that the colitis frequently settles, allowing restoration of bowel continuity at a later date. This therapeutic approach has not had a widespread following.

Crohn's Disease of the Small Intestine

Crohn's disease of the small intestine is a chronic relapsing mucosal and submucosal granulomatous inflammatory disorder affecting any part of the small intestine but with a predilection for the terminal ileum. It occurs alone or in association with colonic disease particularly involving the ascending colon. It heals by fibrosis with the risk of stricture formation; when active it may spread proximally or distally from the site of first involvement and shows a propensity to form enterocutaneous or internal enteric fistulae.

Treatment, Aims and Follow Up

As with colitis, treatment is aimed at suppressing inflammation, controlling symptoms and screening for complications. Follow up is lifelong and should take place in a specialised clinic run by an interested physician. Close co-operation with a gastroenterological surgeon is frequently needed in planning management.

Diagnosis and Assessment

The diagnosis is usually made initially on a barium follow-through or small bowel enema and histological confirmation of the diagnosis occurs when affected gut is resected or when there is associated large bowel disease. After a full history and examination, including sigmoidoscopy, the following baseline investigations are essential: full blood count, differential white cell count, ESR (or other acute phase reactant), blood urea, serum electrolytes, calcium, phosphate, magnesium, iron, total iron binding capacity (or transferrin), folate, vitamin B_{12}, liver function tests, and proteins, stool culture and microscopy and, if not already available, a good barium follow-through (or small bowel enema). A barium enema is necessary to exclude associated colonic Crohn's disease. If there is any suspicion of fat malabsorption, a strict

3-day faecal fat collection is mandatory. A Schilling test and ^{14}C-glycocholate breath test are necessary if there is suspected ileal dysfunction. Bacterial overgrowth is frequently suspected and is investigated with hydrogen or ^{14}C-glycocholate breath test and jejunal or ileal juice aspiration with culture and colony count. Patients with diffuse jejuno-ileal Crohn's disease may show a non-specific malabsorption pattern on barium follow-through and will require a jejunal biopsy, brush border disaccharidase assay and serum immunoglobulins to exclude coeliac disease and Whipple's disease, disaccharidase deficiency, and common variable immune deficiency respectively. In diffuse jejunal Crohn's disease, the jejunal biopsy may show the characteristic histology of Crohn's disease. In difficult cases of ileitis, an ileal biopsy may be necessary. If the stomach or duodenum appear to be involved, upper gastrointestinal endoscopy with biopsy will be indicated. In cases presenting as acute ileitis, *Yersinia* infection will need to be excluded by antibody titres. As with colitis, disease activity is shown by symptoms, fever, raised white cell count, raised ESR, low haemoglobin and low serum albumin.

Management

As in any chronic disorder, treatment involves a large measure of reassurance, support and encouragement and an optimistic attitude from the physician. Patients are treated largely as out-patients, but symptoms such as severe diarrhoea, profound weight loss and malnutrition, and systemic illness and obstruction, as well as symptoms of some of the complications, may require in-patient treatment. It is important when the disease is active that the patient gets plenty of rest, and occasionally patients who cannot or will not rest at home are admitted for this purpose. Where possible, diet should be high protein and high calorie. Patients with frequent subacute obstructive episodes will need a low roughage diet. More serious obstructive episodes may require a period of "drip and suck" in hospital but will rarely require emergency surgery. Severe diarrhoea may require intravenous fluids with potassium and sometimes magnesium supplements. Any anaemia should be characterised and iron, vitamin B_{12} or folic acid given as indicated. If the patient is ill and has a haemoglobin level of less than 10 g/100 ml, transfusion is indicated, provided that all the relevant blood samples have been taken first. Malnourished individuals may benefit from vitamin supplements.

If there is mild active disease, rest and symptomatic treatment for the diarrhoea with codeine phosphate (or equivalent) are often all that is needed. Abdominal pain may respond to anticholinergics or even paracetamol. Further treatment for abdominal pain should be avoided, but if it is necessary, analgesics such as buprenorphine may be used. This drug may add to the constipating effect of the codeine phosphate. More severe disease or persistently active disease may respond to sulphasalazine, although many physicians are unimpressed with it in small intestinal Crohn's disease. If sulphasalazine does not help or if the patient has severe active disease, especially with systemic symptoms, corticosteroids may be indicated. Prednisolone, 40–60 mg per day, is started, and once the symptoms have settled the dose is progressively reduced. In some patients a decrease of the steroid dose can lead to a flare-up of symptoms and weaning off the drug can be difficult or sometimes impossible. Reduction of the dose can be difficult in the presence of continuing disease activity. It is important to remember that steroids are not needed in a majority of symptomatic cases or even in those patients with active disease. Steroids are more likely to be needed in patients with extensive or diffuse small intestinal Crohn's disease, with severe systemic symptoms, and with associated colitis. In addition, steroids may be needed for some of the complications of Crohn's disease (see p. 84). In subacute obstruction, a short course of steroids is worth trying because the obstruction may be caused by inflammatory and oedematous narrowing of the bowel. These patients are likely to have haematological and biochemical evidence of activity. A majority of subacute obstructions are due to fibrotic strictures; the patients have no signs of activity and do not respond to steroids. Steroids are contra-indicated in the presence of abscesses and are of no value in healing fistulae. There is no evidence that steroids prevent relapses or alter the course of the disease. Azathioprine probably has no role in the treatment of Crohn's disease other than as a steroid-sparing agent, although there are anecdotal reports that it may heal fistulae and promote remissions in severely ill patients. Antibiotics are not indicated unless there is an obvious abscess.

Maintenance of nutrition can be difficult in patients with extensive small intestinal disease or resection and in a few, a period of nutritional support is necessary. Enteral nutrition is to be preferred over TPN or elemental diet but occasionally TPN is unavoidable. Bowel rest with TPN may be indicated in an attempt to heal chronic enterocutaneous fistulae.

Patients with small intestinal Crohn's disease may run into problems with malabsorption. The commonest of these is vitamin B_{12} malabsorption due usually to ileal disease or resection but occasionally to a stagnant loop. Folate may be malabsorbed as a result of jejunal disease but may be deficient because of poor dietary intake or excessive utilisation by inflammatory cells. Iron may be malabsorbed as a result of jejunal disease, or deficiency may follow blood loss or poor dietary intake. These problems are treated by the appropriate supplements. Jejunal mucosal involvement may cause disaccharidase deficiencies, lactase usually being the most severely affected. Also primary lactase deficiency may be associated with Crohn's disease. In either situation a lactose-free diet is indicated. Ileal resection or disease may lead to bile salt malabsorption; with less extensive resection or disease, bile salt malabsorption leads to choleraic diarrhoea which is treated with either cholestyramine or Aludrox Gel, both of which bind bile salts. More extensive ileal resection or disease may lead to profound depletion in the total bile salt pool, resulting in a low duodenal and jejunal bile salt concentration. This in turn leads to failure of fat to be formed into micelles with resulting steatorrhoea which can be improved with a low fat diet. Steatorrhoea may follow diffuse jejunal disease and may require a low fat diet. Steatorrhoea may also be caused by bacterial deconjugation of bile salts in a stagnant loop which can result from a stricture or from a bypassed loop following surgery or an entero-enteral fistula. The bacterial overgrowth is treated with antibiotics, usually tetracycline or metronidazole. However, the stagnant loop is treated surgically if possible. In severe cases of steatorrhoea, fat absorption may improve following addition of medium chain triglycerides to the diet. Patients with severe steatorrhoea will need supplements of the fat soluble vitamins, A, D and K.

Long-standing fistulae rarely heal with medical therapy except for the occasional case of spontaneous healing or healing with azathioprine or bowel rest. In contrast, postoperative fistulae may heal without further surgical interference.

As mentioned earlier, follow up is lifelong and requires regular clinical assessment with measurement of haemoglobin, white cell count, ESR and serum albumin to assess activity. Other tests will be repeated as necessary.

Surgery

Surgery in this disorder is an important part of treatment and is complementary to medical treatment. Surgery should not be regarded as the last resort when all attempts at medical management, however heroic, have failed. The patients are often restored to good health much quicker after surgery than after weeks, or even months, of medical management. There is often considerable reluctance to consider operation in patients with Crohn's disease because of the fear of ending up with a patient with the short bowel syndrome. The risk of this has probably been overstated, especially as resections are much more limited now and as the outlook for patients with the short bowel syndrome has considerably improved with modern treatment. If the indications for surgery are present, the future risk of a short bowel syndrome should not deter the operation.

The only absolute indications for surgery are free perforation of the bowel and carcinoma. Relative indications are fistulae and symptomatic strictures without evidence of activity. Subacute obstruction rarely requires urgent surgical intervention and most cases will settle in a day or two on medical therapy. Often surgery may be indicated when the attack has settled down. There are those who feel that resection of diseased small intestine increases the chance of recurrence, especially at the site of anastomosis, but recent evidence suggests that this is not so, although if a resected patient has a recurrence it is most likely to be at the anastomosis. With this in mind, patients with localised but active disease which is impossible to control without steroids will benefit from a resection. Similarly, patients with peri-intestinal abscess will do better after removal of the abscess and resection of the associated diseased gut. Resection of affected gut is always preferable to bypass of the affected gut because of the risk of a stagnant loop with the latter. One exception to this is Crohn's disease of the pyloro-duodenal area, when a gastroenterostomy gives good results. Resection involves removal of the macroscopically affected gut with any associated fistulae or inflammatory tissue; the days of wide excision have long since passed as it is now realised that excision is not curative. Some complications may require surgery and these will be considered later. Patients with acute ileitis may be misdiagnosed as having appendicitis and are operated on. However, the surgeon should avoid appendicectomy and resection of inflamed bowel. A lymph node can be biopsied for histological examination.

Treatment of Complications

Local Complications

Colitis

1. *Peri-anal disease*: This is very common in Crohn's colitis but probably very rare in ulcerative colitis. Haemorrhoids should, if possible, be left alone. If therapy is necessary, anal stretch is usually all that is required. Excision should be avoided if at all possible. Anal skin tags are common, are often mistaken for haemorrhoids and require no treatment. Anal fissures may heal if the colitis settles. If they are troublesome, a gentle anal stretch may be helpful. Peri-anal and ischiorectal abscesses may settle with antibiotics or antimicrobials such as metronidazole in the early stages, although most will require incision and drainage.

Peri-anal fistulae rarely settle with medical treatment or with local surgery such as laying the fistulous track open. However, they can often be left with little upset or discomfort for the patient. The only real treatment that can be offered is proctectomy.

2. *Pseudopolyps* are common in chronic ulcerative colitis but require no treatment.

3. *Toxic megacolon* is seen in both types of colitis, although it also occurs in other types of colonic inflammatory disease. It is defined as total or segmental colonic dilatation in a patient with colitis who is systemically ill with fever, tachycardia, anaemia and neutrophil leucocytosis. If possible, the dilatation is measured on a plain abdominal X-ray at the mid transverse colon, where it is greater than 6 cm in diameter in toxic dilatation. Treatment is urgent and is initiated in the same way as for acute severe colitis (see p. 74). Most clinicians would regard it as an indication for antibiotics. A heterodox view is that toxic dilatation is an indication for colectomy but the orthodox view holds that if there is no significant improvement after 24 hours of medical therapy or if there is deterioration sooner, colectomy should be commenced at once.

4. *Carcinoma* is more common in ulcerative colitis than in Crohn's colitis. It is most frequently seen in those who have long-standing disease, chronically active disease, total disease and/or onset in childhood. Diagnosis is usually made after sigmoidoscopy and barium enema or colonoscopy. As these carcinomas are frequently multiple, treatment is a panproctocolectomy.

5. *Massive haemorrhage*: Medical treatment with replacement blood loss is occasionally successful but this complication frequently requires colectomy.

6. *Strictures* are rare in ulcerative colitis and rarely require treatment. They

are much more common in Crohn's colitis and may need excision although if there is extensive colonic involvement colectomy is advisable.

7. *Perforation* is occasionally seen and also may complicate toxic megacolon. It is always an indication for emergency colectomy.

Crohn's Disease of the Small Intestine

Free perforation and carcinoma are absolute indications for surgery. Obstruction was discussed earlier and rarely requires urgent surgery. Overt bleeding is rarely a problem and can usually be treated medically. Peri-intestinal abscess frequently needs surgery. The treatment of chronic fistulae was also discussed earlier and often the only satisfactory treatment is excision of the fistulous track with resection of the bowel from which the fistula arose. Postoperative fistulae are quite common and frequently heal, although a proportion will become chronic. Peptic ulceration seems to be more common than might be expected and is treated in the usual way.

Systemic Complications

These can be discussed together for colitis and small intestinal Crohn's disease.

Arthritis

Peripheral (usually large) joint arthritis, sacro-iliitis and ankylosing spondylitis may all complicate ulcerative colitis and Crohn's disease.

The arthritis of Crohn's disease tends to run a more benign course which is relatively independent of the bowel disease activity. In contrast, the arthritis of ulcerative colitis can often be severe, with joint destruction, and parallels disease activity. The treatment of arthritis, sacro-iliitis and ankylosing spondylitis is the same as in patients without bowel disease. Steroids may be needed in patients with the arthritis of ulcerative colitis, and severe destructive arthritis may be an indication for panproctocolectomy.

Liver

Patients with ulcerative colitis and Crohn's disease may exhibit a whole range of hepatobiliary disorders—fatty infiltration, pericholangitis, chronic active hepatitis, postnecrotic macronodular cirrhosis, sclerosing cholangitis and bile duct carcinoma. Pericholangitis and fatty infiltration require no treatment. Chronic active hepatitis is treated with steroids for the same indications and in the same way as in patients without inflammatory bowel disease. Cirrhosis requires no treatment unless decompensation appears, which is treated as in other cirrhotic patients. There is no evidence that colectomy reverses these hepatic disorders. Sclerosing cholangitis may involve intra- and/or extrahepatic bile ducts and occasionally may respond to steroids. Usually, however, some attempt at surgical drainage is necessary although this is usually only possible with extrahepatic involvement. In spite of drainage the outlook is frequently poor. Colectomy will not reverse the progress of the disorder. Carcinoma of the bile ducts can be difficult to distinguish from sclerosing cholangitis and diagnosis is usually made after laparotomy. Some form of definitive or, more usually, palliative surgery is necessary. Attacks of cholangitis should be treated with appropriate antibiotics after blood culture.

Cholelithiasis

There is an increased prevalence of gall-stones in patients with ileal resections, ileal disease and ileostomies for both Crohn's and ulcerative colitis as a result of a decrease in the total bile salt pool. If they are troublesome, cholecystectomy is indicated, if necessary with exploration of the common bile duct. Because of the ileal disease, there is no place for dissolution with chenodeoxycholic or ursodeoxycholic acid.

Renal Disorders

Patients with colitis seem to be at risk of pyelonephritis, which is treated in the usual way. Patients with long-standing IBD may be subject to persistent hypokalaemia and resulting hypokalaemic nephropathy. Ureteric obstruction may occur in ulcerative colitis because of a type of retroperitoneal fibrosis. Patients with Crohn's disease, especially involving the terminal ileum, may have ureteric obstruction because of involvement of the ureter in adjacent bowel inflammation or abscess. Treatment of these disorders is surgical. Patients with IBD are at risk of renal calculi. The increased risk of calcium-containing stones may be related to the passage of concentrated urine during episodes of diarrhoea and to increased circulating calcium levels in these patients, which may in turn be related to immobilisation. Excretion of uric acid is higher in IBD patients than in controls and this may lead to urate stone formation, especially if the urine is acid, as frequently occurs in ileostomy patients. Patients with Crohn's disease who have steatorrhoea and an intact colon are liable to hyperoxaluria and resulting oxalate stones. Urinary calculi may require surgical removal but urate stones can sometimes be dissolved by alkalinising the urine and oxalate stones dissolved by reducing hyperoxaluria with a low oxalate diet.

Fistulae from the bowel to the urinary tract are seen in Crohn's disease and require surgical therapy.

Amyloidosis

Patients with ulcerative colitis and Crohn's disease may develop secondary amyloidosis which becomes clinically apparent when the patient develops nephrotic syndrome and renal failure. Treatment is the same as in non-IBD patients and is unsatisfactory. Rarely, secondary amyloid in the small intestine may cause steatorrhoea.

Ocular Complications

Patients with ulcerative colitis and Crohn's disease may suffer from episcleritis or iritis. Rarer ocular problems are keratitis, blepharitis and retinitis. In some patients, the ocular inflammation relapses and remits with bowel disease activity, whereas in others the eye disorders can appear when the bowel disease is quiescent. Most patients with ocular inflammation have other systemic manifestations of IBD. The eye disorders may improve if steroids are given by mouth for bowel inflammation, but if the bowel is quiescent or if oral steroids are not indicated, the eyes can be treated with cycloplegics, mydriatics and topical corticosteroids.

Skin Disorders

1. *Erythema nodosum* may complicate Crohn's disease and occasionally ulcerative colitis. It often requires no treatment but symptoms may be relieved with a non-steroidal anti-inflammatory drug. If symptoms are severe, persist or relapse, oral steroids may be necessary.

2. *Pyoderma gangrenosum* may complicate ulcerative colitis or Crohn's colitis. It is usually associated with severe disease but can be seen in mild cases. It is an indication for steroids, which may control some cases. Persisting and progressive severe pyoderma may be an indication for colectomy, although occasionally even this will not control the disease.

3. *Aphthous ulceration* may be a problem in patients with Crohn's disease and less frequently in ulcerative colitis. It may be associated with disease activity in the bowel in some patients, but this is not invariably the case. Treatment is topical when indicated.

4. *Drug rashes* which may take the form of urticaria, macropapular eruptions or erythema multiforme may be seen and treatment requires withdrawal of the offending drug, often sulphasalazine.

5. *Vasculitis* occurs rarely in ulcerative colitis and requires steroids.

Coagulation Disorders

Bleeding Disorders

Hypoprothrombinaemia is seen in Crohn's disease as a result of vitamin K malabsorption and is easily corrected with supplements. Hypoprothrombinaemia is occasionally seen as a manifestation of hepatic dysfunction in patients with IBD. Treatment is more difficult and may require fresh-frozen plasma infusions. Rarely poor dietary intake of vitamin K may lead to hypoprothrombinaemia in patients with IBD. Disseminated intravascular coagulation may be seen in patients with severe colitis, especially if there is associated septicaemia. It is treated with heparin. Patients with unrelated bleeding disorders are sometimes encountered with colitis and can have a very stormy time.

Thromboembolism

Patients with ulcerative colitis and to a lesser extent Crohn's colitis are at risk from venous thromboembolism, over and above the normal risk in ill bed-bound patients. Increased platelet counts, increased plasma fibrinogen levels and decreased levels of antithrombin III have been found in colitis, all of which would predispose to blood coagulation. Rarely vasculitis will lead to thrombosis. Treatment of established thrombosis consists of intravenous heparin infusion. There is always a risk of colonic bleeding, but the effects of heparin can quickly be reversed if bleeding occurs. Patients with recurring pulmonary emboli may require inferior vena cava ligation and patients with recurring thromboembolism and colonic bleeding may need colectomy.

Inflammatory Bowel Disease and Pregnancy

Women with inflammatory bowel disease who become pregnant will require close monitoring throughout their pregnancy, including the puerperium. Patients will need considerable support and should be managed jointly by an interested physician and an obstetrician. Occasionally a surgeon may need to be involved.

Ulcerative Colitis

There is little evidence that women with ulcerative colitis are anything but normally fertile; therefore the pregnant ulcerative colitic will be a common problem. However, there is no evidence that women with ulcerative colitis are more at risk from abortions, stillbirths, premature births or caesarian sections than healthy women. Nevertheless, ulcerative colitis may sometimes present in pregnancy, usually in the first trimester and very occasionally in the puerperium. In these situations the presentation is often acute and severe and may be life threatening. In patients with known ulcerative colitis whose disease is quiescent at the outset of pregnancy, there seems to be an increased risk of relapse, especially during the first trimester and the puerperium, although a recent study from Oxford suggests that this may not be so. If the disease is active at the onset, there is a high risk of continuing symptoms and even deterioration, but in some the colitis may actually improve. Severe colitis at the onset of pregnancy reduces the chance of a normal outcome. Patients with an ileostomy and panproctocolectomy usually have no problems, although ileostomy prolapse may sometimes occur.

   Treatment of ulcerative colitis in pregnancy is the same as in non-pregnant patients. There is no evidence that steroids or sulphasalazine are harmful to the foetus. However, X-rays should be avoided during the first trimester and sigmoidoscopy and rectal therapy should be avoided if possible during the second and third trimesters. If the patient is ill, X-rays and sigmoidoscopy should not be withheld. Patients are particularly liable to iron deficiency. Indications for colectomy are the same as in non-pregnant patients and colectomy should not be delayed in severe acute colitis if it would be indicated in normal circumstances. There is virtually no indication for therapeutic abortion in the management of the pregnant ulcerative colitic.

Crohn's Disease

Women with Crohn's disease are more likely to be infertile or subfertile than healthy women. Women with Crohn's colitis are more likely to have problems than patients with small intestinal Crohn's disease. Subfertility is often associated with disease activity and/or malabsorption or malnutrition and may improve as the disease becomes quiescent or if malabsorption and malnutrition are appropriately treated.

There is little evidence that Crohn's disease has an adverse effect on the pregnancy, and the outcome is usually good. It is very rare for Crohn's disease to present during pregnancy or the puerperium. Women with inactive Crohn's disease at the start of pregnancy usually do well, although relapse is possible, especially in the puerperium. Women with active disease at the start may continue with symptoms and may deteriorate during the pregnancy, but other cases remit.

Treatment is the same as in non-pregnant females, although surgery in small intestinal Crohn's disease tends to be avoided if at all possible until after the pregnancy.

Inflammatory Bowel Disease in the Elderly

The important consideration here is to remember that both ulcerative colitis and Crohn's disease, especially colitis, can occur in the elderly, for it is easy to ascribe the symptoms to other causes. Therefore, sigmoidoscopy and rectal biopsy as well as a barium enema are mandatory in bloody diarrhoea of the elderly. Treatment is the same as in younger patients and surgery should follow on the same indications. If colectomy is indicated, it should be a total one; it is tempting to try to get away with a lesser procedure such as a partial colectomy and colostomy but this is frequently disastrous. Elderly patients may have coexisting disease such as hypertension, diabetes mellitus or osteoporosis; these conditions may be aggravated by corticosteroids and the patients often cannot retain enemata. Some elderly patients often cannot or will not eat a sufficient diet and can be easily given nutritional support with enteral feeding.

Inflammatory Bowel Disease in Childhood

Inflammatory bowel disease presenting in children is an increasingly recognised problem and requires considerable patience and clinical skill on the part of the paediatric gastroenterologist. Patients and their parents require considerable reassurance and support, and management is often rendered difficult by a negative and resentful attitude on the part of the adolescent patient whose life may be considerably hampered by the disease and/or its treatment.

Ulcerative Colitis

Ulcerative colitis is a major problem because it tends to have an acute onset with total involvement of the bowel and seems to run a more chronic course than in most adults. It results in nutritional and growth problems as well as emotional problems. Moreover the risk of developing carcinoma in later life seems to be greater if onset is in childhood. As well as the usual symptoms of ulcerative colitis, children may present with anaemia, extracolonic complications or growth failure. History and full examination, including sigmoidoscopy, are followed by the same baseline investigations as in adults. Treatment is the same as in adults, but withdrawal of corticosteroids without relapse can be more difficult than in adults so long-term steroid treatment with resultant growth problems is all too common. Indications for colectomy are the same as in adults and colectomy should not be postponed because of the child's age. Children usually adjust well to an ileostomy. An indication for colectomy in children is frequently the necessity for high dose steroid therapy, leading to growth retardation, susceptibility to infections, osteoporosis and myopathy. After a colectomy, these children do very much better. Colectomy should also be considered as an alternative form of therapy, for the long-term outlook for children with ulcerative colitis is not good, especially because of the cancer risk.

Crohn's Disease

Crohn's disease can affect any part of the bowel in children just as it can in adults, although it frequently seems to be more florid in the former. It provides a considerable challenge to the paediatric gastroenterologist and paediatric surgeon and provides many of the problems already discussed in ulcerative colitis in childhood. Management of small intestinal Crohn's disease and Crohn's colitis is largely the same as in adults. Steroids are often needed to suppress inflammatory activity and frequently lead to problems, the worst of which is growth failure. Therefore surgery should be considered early in this situation, but unlike the situation in childhood ulcerative colitis, resection may not always be possible because of the distribution or extent of disease. In spite of the severe effects of steroids on growing children, some paediatricians claim that every child with Crohn's disease should be started on steroids. This would seem a terrible and potentially disastrous attitude, for children, like adults, frequently require no more than symptomatic treatment with appropriate nutritional supplements, including haematinics. A problem of Crohn's disease itself is also growth failure, which is most often seen in diffuse small intestinal disease. This is potentially reversible and improves after resection of the diseased tissue. In situations where this is impossible, growth spurts have been achieved with long periods of TPN.

Further Reading

Cooke WT, Allan RN (1980) Inflammatory bowel disease. In: Bouchier IAD (ed) Recent advances in gastroenterology, vol 4. Churchill Livingstone, Edinburgh London New York, pp 117–146

Cooke WT, Mallas E, Prior P, Allan RN (1980) Crohn's disease: cause, treatment and long term prognosis. Q J Med 49: 363–384

Dyer NH (1975) Ulcerative colitis and Crohn's disease. In: Anderson CM, Burke V (eds) Paediatric gastroenterology. Blackwell, Oxford, pp 411–453

Farmer RG (ed) (1980) Inflammatory bowel disease. Clin Gastroenterol 9: 229–481

Fielding JF (1976) Inflammatory bowel disease and pregnancy. Br J Hosp Med 4: 345–352

Kirsner JB, Shorter RG (eds) (1980) Inflammatory bowel disease, 2nd edn. Lea and Febiger, Philadelphia

Lennard-Jones JE, Singleton JW (1981) The azathioprine controversy. Dig Dis Sci 26: 364–371

6 The Irritable Bowel Syndrome and Diverticular Disease

A. P. Manning

Introduction

Of all patients referred to a gastroenterology clinic, nearly half will have no organic cause found on investigation to explain their symptoms. If they complain of disturbances of bowel habit or abdominal pain, or both, then a diagnosis of irritable bowel syndrome (IBS) may be made. Others with similar symptoms will be found to have colonic diverticula. This chapter deals with these two groups of patients.

Irritable bowel syndrome is a common diagnosis in Western Europe and North American practice. Accurate prevalence data are not available as diagnostic criteria are imprecise. It has been suggested, however, that about 14% of apparently healthy Britons have symptoms suggestive of IBS. The disorder presents more commonly in females and, although it can occur at any age, characteristically affects those in the third and fourth decade.

Diverticular disease has a similar geographical distribution to IBS. Its prevalence increases with age, 40% of those over 70 years having colonic diverticula. However, only a minority of those with diverticula develop relevant symptoms.

Pathophysiology

Irritable bowel syndrome is regarded as a disorder of intestinal motility. Recordings of intestinal motor activity are difficult to interpret, but those of IBS patients show differences from "normal" controls in both small and large bowel.

Most recording techniques register peaks of increased pressure or muscle activity during segmental contraction of the bowel. IBS patients with constipation and with pain tend to have an increased frequency and amplitude of these peaks compared with controls, whereas patients with diarrhoea tend to have fewer peaks. Some patients may feel pain coincident with recorded pressure peaks, the hypothesis being that pain results from distension proximal to an area of intense segmenting contraction represented by the peaks.

Normal subjects have an increase in colonic motor activity after meals. IBS patients with postprandial symptoms may have an exaggerated activity response to food associated with pain.

Patients with IBS have abnormal motility responses to various other stimuli. Emotional stress, traditionally regarded as a major aetiological factor in IBS, is said to increase the segmenting activity in patients complaining mainly of pain and constipation, but to decrease the segmenting activity in those complaining mainly of diarrhoea. IBS patients also have a marked colonic motility response to injected cholinergic agents, such as neostigmine.

The cause of these abnormal motor responses in IBS is unclear. The myoelectric potentials in the sigmoid colon of patients have been recorded and most groups report them as being abnormal in IBS. In this condition there appears to be an abnormal proportion of slow wave activity at a frequency of three cycles per minute. This abnormality has been found in patients complaining of diarrhoea and in patients complaining of constipation, during both remissions and relapses. The relationship between this apparently consistent abnormality and the various changes in motor activity is not understood.

Some studies have indicated that in IBS the colon is more sensitive to painful stimuli than normal. If a balloon is distended in the sigmoid colon, pain is felt at lower inflation volumes in IBS patients than in control subjects.

In summary, therefore, IBS patients have abnormalities in the recorded myoelectric and motor activities of the bowel although there is no unifying hypothesis to relate all these measurements to symptoms. The adverse effects of these abnormal motor activities seem to be compounded by an undue sensitivity of the bowel wall to distension.

Diverticular disease is characterised both by the presence of diverticula and by an abnormal thickening of the colonic musculature with resulting luminal narrowing. These changes are characteristically seen in the sigmoid and descending colons. Those patients with symptoms are thought to have abnormalities of colonic motor activity similar to those seen in IBS. Recording devices in the sigmoid colon record peaks of intraluminal pressure coincident with segmental contraction. These peaks may be accentuated after food or cholinergic agents. It has been established that the symptoms of uncomplicated diverticular disease are related to the muscle abnormality rather than the diverticula themselves.

Exacerbating Factors

Many patients with IBS, and some with diverticular disease, experience worsening of their symptoms during times of emotional stress. This may be but an exaggeration of the intestinal upset experienced by most people before, for example, an examination or public-speaking engagement. Counselling patients of the possibility of this occurrence may allay their anxiety if symptoms increase during times of stress.

Some patients with these disorders will experience symptoms after certain foods. Those items implicated vary from patient to patient but common ones are fatty foods, onions, citrus fruits and beer. Patients should know from experience which foods to avoid initially but when symptoms are controlled on treatment, these foods can be cautiously reintroduced.

General Management

The essential first step in the management of IBS is to make the diagnosis using the minimum of special tests. A series of unnecessary negative investigations only reinforces the patient's impression of obscure organic disease. The diagnosis having been made confidently, the patient can be reassured and treatment started.

Diverticular disease is a common finding on barium enema examination, especially in older people. It is therefore important to determine whether the patient's symptoms are compatible with the radiological findings. For example, occult gastrointestinal bleeding in a patient with diverticular disease should be further investigated as diverticula do not commonly cause this type of bleeding. Again, if the patient's symptoms are attributable to demonstrated diverticular disease, treatment can be started.

A proportion of patients presenting with the symptoms of IBS may be suffering from clinical anxiety or depression or both. In some, this may be alleviated by strong reassurance. In the minority, in whom the psychological symptoms are predominant, appropriate psychotropic medications or formal psychotherapy may be helpful.

Currently, the mainstay of treatment for IBS and for uncomplicated diverticular disease is a high-fibre diet. It is a widely held belief, based mainly on epidemiological evidence, that a fibre-depleted diet is instrumental in the aetiology of both conditions. In some, but not all, clinical trials a high-fibre diet has been shown to alleviate symptoms and to reduce colonic intraluminal pressures. In practice such a diet should include wholemeal bread, the use of wholemeal flour in cooking, brown rice rather than white and ample fresh fruits and vegetables.

Drug treatment need be advised only if symptoms are still troublesome after a fair trial of a high-fibre diet lasting 6–8 weeks or are initially severe.

Drug Treatment

The types of drug most commonly used in IBS and uncomplicated diverticular disease are stool bulking agents and "antispasmodics". Occasionally other laxatives or anti-diarrhoeal agents are used as appropriate for temporary symptomatic relief.

Stool Bulking Agents

Stool bulking agents increase stool volume and some have been shown to reduce colonic intraluminal pressures in these disorders. Several clinical trials have demonstrated significant improvement in symptoms with these preparations.

Unprocessed wheat bran is probably the bulking agent of choice in most patients. It is cheap, adaptable to the high-fibre diet and readily obtainable without a doctor's prescription. Its action is incompletely understood but is only partly due to its water-holding capacity. It should be introduced in a small dose, for example one teaspoon twice daily, which can be increased gradually until symptomatic relief is obtained. Patients should be warned to expect increased bloating sensations initially which are self-limiting on continuing to take bran. Its major drawback is that some patients find bran unpalatable. It has few other potential adverse effects. It does increase faecal losses of calcium, phosphorus, magnesium and zinc although there is no evidence that this is significant in the clinical context.

Other bulking agents are either derived from the fibrous components of other plant materials or are semi-synthetic polysaccharides. *Sterculia* and ispaghula are examples of the former type and methyl-cellulose of the latter. The choice between these preparations depends upon their palatability for the individual patient, there probably being little to choose between their clinical efficacy. They have few adverse effects. They all tend to increase any sensation of bloating early in treatment and patients should be told to expect this. There have been isolated case reports of intestinal obstruction due to impaction of an intraluminal mass of bulking agent. These patients usually have some structural abnormality of the gastrointestinal tract or have been consuming excessively large quantities of the substance.

"Antispasmodics"

Colonic hypermotility, as inferred from studies of colonic motor activity and from radiology, is the rationale for the use of antispasmodic drugs in both IBS and diverticular disease.

Traditionally, anticholinergic agents have been used in these conditions but they have actions on organ systems other than the gut. Few of these drugs have been tested by rigorously controlled clinical trials. In fairness, such trials are difficult to carry out in conditions such as these, where characteristically symptoms fluctuate and there is no unequivocal end-point; nobody dies of IBS. A further problem with testing these, and other, compounds is that there may be up to a 35% placebo response in IBS, at least in the short term.

Many anticholinergic agents have been used in these conditions with claims of benefit. These include atropine, hyoscine compounds, mepenzolate, clidinium and dicyclomine. A major drawback of their use is the significant incidence of adverse effects. These commonly involve dryness of the mouth and blurring of vision and, more importantly, in the older patient with diverticular disease they may precipitate glaucoma and urinary retention.

An antispasmodic drug which is not anticholinergic and is claimed to act directly on colonic muscle is mebeverine. Clinical studies suggest its superiority to placebo in IBS. Its lack of anticholinergic side-effects has ensured its wide use in these disorders.

Another preparation currently in favour for IBS is peppermint oil. This has been shown in one study to relax gut muscle and to be preferred to placebo by IBS patients. Its major side-effect, that of relaxing the lower oesophageal sphincter and causing gastro-oesophageal reflux, may be minimised by its formulation in enteric-coated capsules.

Drug Combinations

Not unexpectedly in conditions with inconsistent responses to various treatments, regimes have been formulated to combine various agents, with reported benefit. For example, one study testing various combinations of agents reported the most effective in IBS patients to be ispaghula, fluphenazine/nortriptyline mixture and mebeverine.

In summarising this section it may be said that in those patients not responding to a high-fibre diet alone a stool bulking agent acceptable to the patient should be used. If this fails to provide consistent relief of symptoms then an antispasmodic drug may be added, its choice being governed by its incidence of side-effects.

Complications and Surgical Treatment

There is no indication for surgical treatment in IBS. Indeed, it may be said that surgery is a complication of IBS. It is likely that many normal appendices and asymptomatic gall-stones are removed for symptoms actually caused by IBS. Obviously, these symptoms recur within months of the unnecessary operation.

Debate continues as to whether diverticular disease itself is a complication of long-standing IBS. The conditions have an identical geographical distribution and similar, if not identical, pathophysiological features. In one follow-up study of IBS patients, more were said to develop diverticula than would be expected in a normal population. However, few patients presenting with symptomatic diverticular disease will recall chronic symptoms that suggest IBS earlier in life.

Only a small proportion of patients with diverticular disease require operation. Some patients with intractable symptoms and much colonic muscle hypertrophy demonstrated radiologically may undergo elective surgery.

Segmental resection is the usual operative procedure although sigmoid longitudinal myotomy has had a vogue. Studies have suggested a high incidence of recurrent symptoms after these operations although there are suggestions that a high-fibre diet may reduce this.

Most operations for diverticular disease are performed for complications of the condition. It is true to say that the symptoms of diverticular disease are due to the muscle abnormality but the complications are related to the diverticula themselves.

Probably the commonest complication is diverticulitis, a peri-colonic inflammation consequent upon microperforation of a diverticulum. This causes left iliac pain along with the concomitants of inflammation, fever, leucocytosis and a palpable, tender mass. Treatment is usually conservative with bed rest and fluids; antibiotics are often added on empirical grounds. If the inflammation does not settle, becomes more widespread or is recurrent, then operative intervention may be called for.

Other inflammatory conditions consequent upon the perforation of a diverticulum include abscess formation, generalised peritonitis and fistula formation, usually to the bladder. These complications are usually an indication for surgical management. Various operations have been devised, none achieving universal acceptance, but often entailing a temporary defunctioning colostomy. The operative management of the condition has been extensively reviewed elsewhere (see "Further Reading").

The other noteworthy complication of diverticular disease is colonic haemorrhage. Classically this results in moderate blood loss. It is usually self-limiting and rarely requires more than the conservative measures of bed rest and blood transfusion. A minority of patients continue to bleed so as to require resective surgery. It is important in these cases to identify the source of the haemorrhage pre-operatively by selective angiography. This is essential in order to define the area for resection and to exclude bleeding from angiodysplastic lesions in the right colon, which is not uncommon in elderly patients.

Further Reading

Almy TP, Howell DA (1980) Diverticular disease of the colon. N Engl J Med 302: 324–331
Ivey KJ (1975) Are anticholinergics of use in the irritable colon syndrome? Gastroenterology 68: 1300–1307
Rees WD, Evans BK, Rhodes J (1979) Treating irritable bowel syndrome with peppermint oil. Br Med J II: 835–836
Ritchie JA, Truelove SC (1980) Comparisons of various treatments for irritable bowel syndrome. Br Med J 281: 1317–1319
Smith AN (ed) (1975) Diverticular disease. Clin Gastroenterol 4(1) Saunders, London Philadelphia Toronto
Thompson WG (1979) The irritable gut. University Park Press, Baltimore

7 Diseases of the Biliary System

K. W. Heaton

Introduction

This chapter is concerned only with the diseases of the biliary system which are likely to present to the physician. It does not deal with tumours of the gall bladder and bile ducts since these are essentially surgical diseases, nor with adenomyosis and cholesterolosis of the gall bladder since these have little if any clinical significance.

By far the most important disease affecting the biliary system is cholelithiasis or gall-stones. It is probably the commonest disease affecting the digestive apparatus. Autopsy surveys in urban communities around the world reveal that cholelithiasis is rare in young adult life but becomes steadily commoner with age so that by the age of 70 it is present in 30%–60% of women. In men it is about half as common. Gall-stones are much commoner in obese people, and there are significant associations with diabetes, hypertriglyceridaemia, hiatus hernia and, probably, diverticular disease.

Pathophysiology of Gall-stones

In western civilisation most gall-stones are composed mainly of crystalline cholesterol and a few are pure cholesterol. The other crystalline components are chiefly calcium salts, including carbonate, phosphate, palmitate and bilirubinate, and occasionally these predominate. Pigment stones consist mainly of unidentified amorphous material. The pathogenesis of non-cholesterol stones is still obscure, whereas that of cholesterol stones is quite well understood.

In bile, cholesterol is solubilised in micelles of bile acids and phospholipids. Hepatic bile—that is, bile freshly secreted into the canaliculi—is supersaturated with cholesterol if the rate of cholesterol secretion is excessive and/or the rate of bile acid and phospholipid secretion is inadequate. The bile from which gall-stones form is the bile which is diverted into the gall bladder as digestion nears completion, to be retained and concentrated there until the next meal. In this process, the bile acid pool, which is constantly moving round the enterohepatic circulation during digestion, is largely sequestered in the gall bladder. Hence the main determinant of the bile acid (and, secondarily, phospholipid) content of the relaxed gall bladder is the size of the bile-acid pool. In patients with gall-stones the bile acid pool is reduced from the normal mean of 3 g to 1.5–2.0 g. Most workers believe that, except in some very obese people, this is a major factor in the production of supersaturated gall bladder bile.

The cause of the small bile acid pool has not been established, but many workers believe it is due to suppression of hepatic bile acid synthesis. The major rate-limiting enzyme in this synthesis, cholesterol 7α-hydroxylase, is less active in the livers of patients with gall-stones than in controls. The cause of this is not clear and it is not even known whether the difference is congenital or acquired.

Cholesterol secretion into bile is excessive in many patients with gall-stones, especially those who are obese. It is also excessive in many obese people without gall-stones but they tend to have normal or large bile acid pools. Cholesterol secretion is probably determined, at least in part, by the rate of cholesterol synthesis, and the enzyme which controls the rate of cholesterol synthesis, HMG-CoA-reductase, seems to be over-active in the livers of patients with gall-stones. This enzyme is stimulated by insulin and its activity is increased in obesity.

Thus, the two metabolic abnormalities of patients with gall-stones—excessive secretion of cholesterol and a small bile-acid pool—are probably due to enhanced synthesis of cholesterol and suppressed synthesis of bile acids respectively.

In westernised countries many people *without* gall-stones have supersaturated gall bladder bile, which implies that additional factors are necessary. Possible factors are nucleating agents, which might be bacteria or desquamated cells, and deficiency of substances which inhibit crystal growth. The gall bladder may play a part, but otherwise it is uncertain whether it has a role in the formation of gall-stones beyond acting as a quiet cul-de-sac in which there is time for crystals to precipitate, grow and stick together. The fact that it concentrates bile is not necessarily relevant, as the cholesterol-solubilising capacity of a bile acid–phospholipid mixture increases as it becomes more concentrated.

The growth of a gall-stone is believed to represent the result of a balance between growth and spontaneous dissolution, two processes which occur at different rates at different times.

Gall-stones cause symptoms only when they obstruct a duct. Obstruction of the cystic duct leads to biliary colic or, if prolonged, acute cholecystitis. Obstruction of the common bile duct leads to cholestatic jaundice or ascending cholangitis or both. Acute pancreatitis is often accompanied by the passage of a stone through the ampulla of Vater and is presumably due to impaired drainage of pancreatic secretions or to reflux of duodenal contents through a damaged sphincter of Vater.

The traditional belief that gall-stones cause flatulent dyspepsia has been disproved by several surveys, but dies hard.

Most gall-stones are asymptomatic. Autopsy surveys indicate that up to 75% of cases are unsuspected in life, but silent stones are probably commoner in elderly people than in those who are younger. On prolonged follow up, silent stones do eventually cause severe symptoms in a proportion of cases, but the figure may be as low as 20%.

Therapeutic Principles

The first decision to be taken is whether to treat at all. When gall bladder calculi are an incidental finding in an elderly patient or in someone for whom anaesthesia and surgery are unusually dangerous, they can reasonably be left alone. At the other extreme, the patient should of course be treated if gall-stones are causing severe biliary colic. Stones in the bile ducts should always be treated even if they are asymptomatic. Patients who are fit for surgery but who have few if any symptoms should have the three options explained to them—wait and see, surgery or drugs.

Having decided to treat, the physician must then decide between medical and surgical treatment. Surgery is swift and highly effective in all cases, regardless of the type and site of stone. However, it involves hospital admission, some pain and at least 6 weeks off work. Complications are uncommon after cholecystectomy but can be serious. Treatment fails, in the sense that common duct stones are left behind in about 10% of cases requiring exploration of the common bile duct. Deaths are rare, but do occur.

Medical treatment is attractive because it is completely safe, as far as is known, and completely painless. It avoids admission to hospital and time off work. It is also logical, since cholelithiasis is, in origin at least, a metabolic disease, not a mechanical one. However, medical treatment is not always effective. It is completely ineffective with calcified or radio-opaque stones even when there is only a thin layer of calcium salts. It is completely ineffective for gall bladder stones when the gall bladder is "non-functioning", that is, it fails to opacify on oral cholecystography. It is relatively ineffective when stones are larger than 15 mm diameter; these seldom dissolve and, if they do, it can take more than 2 years.

Other disadvantages of medical treatment are:

1. Even in properly selected cases, where small radiolucent stones occupy a functioning gall bladder, there is at best an 80% success rate. This is because only 80% of radiolucent stones are composed predominantly of cholesterol; some "pigment" stones are radiolucent. The real success rate is always considerably lower than 80% because some patients drop out. With oral drug treatment of common duct stones the success rate is, at best, 50% and the risk of complications is high.

2. Treatment usually takes between 1 and 2 years. During this time the patient must visit the hospital at least 7–13 times.

3. There is appreciable radiation exposure from repeated cholecystograms.

4. Recurrence of gall-stones occurs in up to 70% of patients in the first few years after treatment is stopped.

5. Because of the risk of recurrence the patient can never be considered cured and must to the end of her life think of herself as needing medical attention like a diabetic or hypertensive patient.

6. With chenodeoxycholic acid treatment, diarrhoea can be annoying or even disabling.

Ideally, suitability for treatment should be confirmed by duodenal intubation and aspiration of gall bladder bile for analysis of cholesterol saturation. The presence of unsaturated bile would reveal the 20% of patients with pigment-rich stones, who could then be excluded, thus saving much time and expense. However, this is only practicable in academic departments which have bile analysis as an established research technique. Moreover, duodenal intubation is uncomfortable for some patients. The mere thought of it might deter some patients from agreeing to be treated.

The attractions of medical treatment are obvious to the patient. Its disadvantages are not at all obvious and should be carefully explained before a decision to treat medically is taken. The decision is one to be taken by the patient as much as by the doctor.

The only clear-cut indication for medical treatment is unfitness for anaesthesia and abdominal surgery. On humanitarian grounds, a morbid fear of surgery may be considered a relative indication. Otherwise, it is a case of balancing the pros and cons. Ideally, cost should influence the decision but, under the National Health Service, it is impossible to make precise estimates of the cost of medical or surgical treatment regimes. Probably there is no great difference in this case.

Exacerbating Factors

Excess body weight promotes the secretion of cholesterol into bile and obese people require larger doses of chenodeoxycholic acid—possibly 20 mg/kg body weight per day—to obtain unsaturated bile. It may be a high energy (calorie) intake which is the exacerbating factor since, if obese subjects eat a low energy diet, they respond to the normal dose of 15 mg/kg per day, even before they have lost weight. There is some evidence that inclusion of refined carbohydrates (especially sugar and white flour) in the diet increases the cholesterol saturation of bile. It also elevates energy intake. Whether excluding refined carbohydrates would enhance the effect of gall-stone-dissolving agents remains to be seen. The role of dietary fat is even more uncertain. In practice, limitation of fat and refined carbohydrate is an integral part of most reducing diets.

Treatment with oestrogens and with clofibrate increases the cholesterol saturation of bile and probably favours gall-stone formation. These effects have not been shown with the low dose of oestrogen used in most current contraceptive pills, nor has it been shown that the effect of bile acid treatment is reduced by oestrogen or clofibrate treatment. However, it makes good sense to avoid these drugs as far as possible during medical treatment of gall-stones.

General Management

A low-fat diet has a time-honoured place in the symptomatic treatment of patients with gall-stones. It is widely and plausibly believed to relieve flatulent dyspepsia and even to reduce the frequency of biliary colic. Its value has never been subjected to controlled trials but it is harmless and there seems no reason to discontinue the practice, provided the patient finds it helpful.

Weight reduction is often recommended to make surgery safer in obese patients. It is also an important adjunct to medical treatment since it probably increases its effect or allows a smaller dose of drugs to be given. In Bristol we routinely advise a slimming diet to all overweight gall-stone patients on bile acid treatment. This may be responsible for the relatively low recurrence rate (25%). However, heavy emphasis on slimming may discourage some patients and cause them to abandon treatment.

A diet low in cholesterol and saturated fat has been recommended by some workers, but the evidence that it helps bile acid treatment is limited and more data are needed before it can be generally recommended.

Drug Treatment of Gall-stones

The drugs which have proven ability to dissolve gall-stones are chenodeoxycholic acid, ursodeoxycholic acid and a mixture of plant terpenes marketed as Rowachol.

Chenodeoxycholic Acid (CDCA)

Physiology

Chenodeoxycholic acid is not really a drug but a natural component of the body. In man the bile acid pool consists of about 1 g CDCA and 1.3 g cholic acid, which are the two primary bile acids synthesised in the liver from cholesterol, together with about 0.5 g deoxycholic acid, which is a secondary bile acid derived from bacterial dehydroxylation of cholic acid in the colon. There are also trace amounts of lithocholic acid, which is the equivalent metabolite of CDCA (Fig. 1).

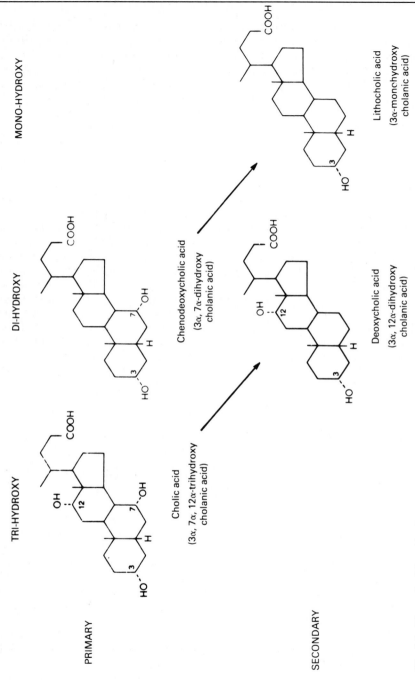

Fig. 7.1. The major bile acids of man

The bile acid pool is efficiently conserved by an enterohepatic circulation. The pool is reabsorbed mainly in the terminal ileum and, if the gall bladder is contracted and the sphincter of Oddi is relaxed, as during digestion, the bile acid pool re-enters the duodenum within an hour or two. During an average day the pool circulates six to ten times, which means that the intestine receives about 20 g of natural detergent every day. Of this, only 0.3–0.5 g escapes in the faeces, to be promptly replaced by newly synthesised bile acid. Lithocholic acid is conserved less well than the other three bile acids because when it reaches the liver it is sulphated to a more polar substance which is poorly reabsorbed.

Mode of Action

When CDCA treatment was introduced in 1971 it was thought to work by expanding the bile acid pool. However, it was soon found that feeding cholic acid also expands the pool but does not render bile less saturated with cholesterol. Moreover, pool expansion should be complete within 2 or 3 days of starting CDCA at, say 1 g per day, whereas the fall in bile saturation continues for 10–20 days. This suggests a more subtle metabolic rearrangement. It has been clearly shown that CDCA has two relevant effects on hepatic cholesterol metabolism. It reduces the secretion of cholesterol into bile by about 40% and it suppresses the activity of the rate-limiting enzyme for cholesterol synthesis (HMG–CoA reductase) by a similar amount. It is tempting to conclude, as many have done, that CDCA works thus:

Less cholesterol synthesised in liver
$\downarrow$

Less cholesterol secreted into bile
$\downarrow$

Less saturated bile

However, it is probably not as simple as this because cholesterol in bile is derived mainly from the catabolism of lipoproteins rather than from newly synthesised material.

Dosage

Dose-response curves have shown that to obtain consistently unsaturated bile it is necessary to take at least 15 mg/kg body weight per day. For the average female patient this amounts to 1000 mg a day, which can be taken as four capsules of 250 mg. Capsules of 125 mg are also available. There is quite good evidence that a given daily dose of CDCA is more effective if taken altogether at bedtime than if taken in divided doses through the day. This is also easier for the patient to remember.

When she is started on CDCA, the patient should be warned about the possibility of diarrhoea and advised to reduce the dose by half if it occurs. She should then build up the dose gradually to the maximum tolerated. If diarrhoea recurs the following options are available: (a) add an anti-diarrhoeal agent, (b) change to ursodeoxycholic acid (UDCA) and, possibly, (c) change to a mixture of CDCA and UDCA or of CDCA and Rowachol (see p. 106).

Toxic Effects

The only proven toxic effect is diarrhoea. This occurs to an annoying extent in up to 20% of patients on 15 mg/kg per day and to a minor extent in about half the remainder. Often it is intermittent. In a few cases there is colic. The mechanism for loose stools is almost certainly the cathartic effect of unabsorbed dihydroxy bile acids spilling into the colon.

A rise in plasma aspartate aminotransferase concentration to two or three times the upper limit of normal occurs within the first few weeks in about 30% of patients. This is transient and is not associated with any other abnormality of liver function. Liver biopsies during CDCA treatment have shown no detectable changes on light microscopy and only minor changes of doubtful significance on electron microscopy. Significant hepatotoxicity almost certainly does not occur in man. It does occur in many other species, probably because they are less efficient at sulphating and so ridding themselves of lithocholic acid, a highly toxic material.

Other Metabolic Effects

There is often a fall in the fasting plasma triglyceride concentration and in hypertriglyceridaemic patients this can be substantial. Plasma cholesterol does not change. There were early fears that total body cholesterol would rise, due to the depression of bile acid synthesis which is the major catabolic pathway of cholesterol. This has not been found to occur, but appropriate studies are admittedly few in number. There has been one report of a slight but consistent rise in fasting plasma glucose and of a consistent fall in plasma D-glutamyl transferase, but the significance of these changes is unclear.

Resistance

A few patients, obese or not, fail to show the expected fall in the cholesterol saturation of bile. The reason is uncertain, but the existence of this phenomenon suggests that, when possible, duodenal intubation and bile analysis should be performed after, say, 1 month's treatment to check drug action.

Monitoring Treatment

There is no need to do regular liver function tests. Patients should be seen initially within 2–4 weeks to determine whether diarrhoea is a problem but thereafter, in straightforward cases, they can be seen every 3 months. When the stones are very small, an oral cholecystogram can reasonably be obtained after 3 months' treatment. Otherwise, cholecystograms should be performed at 6-monthly intervals until complete dissolution has occurred. No preliminary film is necessary. When a clear cholecystogram is obtained, treatment should be continued for 2 or 3 months to ensure the complete disappearance of any very small, undetectable stones. Where good ultrasonography is available this can be used to supplement or partially replace cholecystography. Treatment should probably be stopped if, despite good compliance, bed-time dosing and adherence to a slimming diet, three consecutive cholecystograms show no change in the size of stones.

After successful treatment it is probably wise to arrange an annual cholecystogram or ultrasonogram, at least for 3 years.

Recurrence

Radiologically detectable recurrence can be expected to occur eventually in up to 70% of patients unless special measures are taken. Most recurrences take place during the first year. A co-operative study is under way in five British centres to discover whether recurrence can be prevented by (a) a diet low in refined carbohydrate and enriched with bran and (b) continuous low-dose ursodeoxycholic acid therapy.

Ursodeoxycholic Acid (UDCA)

This interesting drug shows many resemblances to CDCA but also some important and valuable differences. It became available in the U.K. in 1981 but has been used extensively in Japan since 1975.

Physiology

Ursodeoxycholic acid is chemically identical with CDCA except that the 7-hydroxyl group is in the β instead of the α configuration (Fig. 2). It is present in trace amounts in some people's bile and increases when they are fed CDCA. This is because it is derived from CDCA by bacterial dehydrogenation in the colon followed, after absorption, by oxidation in the liver (Fig. 2). This is a two-way process so that when radio-labelled UDCA is fed, bile comes to contain some labelled CDCA. Like CDCA, UDCA can be dehydroxylated to lithocholic acid. UDCA is less soluble than CDCA and less efficient at forming micelles. However, it circulates enterohepatically in the same way.

Mode of Action

The mode of action is basically the same as with CDCA but UDCA may be more effective at expanding the bile acid pool. This could help to explain its greater potency in desaturating bile.

Dosage

Dose-response curves show that it is necessary to take only 8–10 mg/kg per day to obtain consistently unsaturated bile. It is available in 150-mg capsules (e.g. Destolit). The effect of bedtime dosing is unknown.

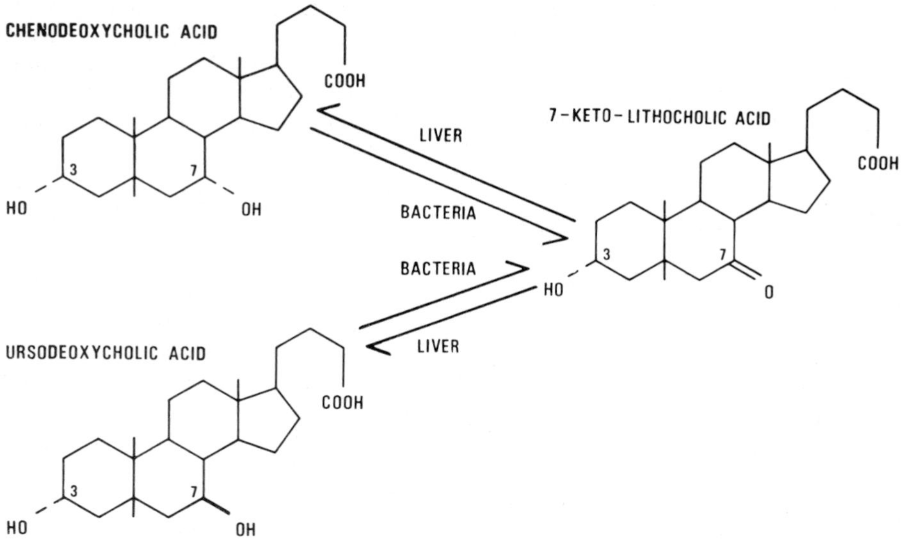

Fig. 7.2. Chenodeoxycholic and ursodeoxycholic acids, and their intermediate metabolite 7-keto-lithocholic acid

Toxic Effects

The great advantage of UDCA is that it does not cause diarrhoea. This is apparently because it differs from CDCA (and deoxycholic acid) in not causing the colonic mucosa to secrete water and electrolytes. Furthermore, UDCA does not lead to elevation of plasma transaminases, even at a dose of 15 mg/kg per day.

Other Features

Other metabolic effects are similar to those of CDCA.
Resistance has not so far been reported.
Monitoring should be the same as with CDCA.
The cost of UDCA is greater than that of CDCA (from which it is manufactured) but this is offset by its lower dosage.

Rowachol

This is a proprietary mixture of menthol and smaller amounts of five other plant terpenes–pinene, menthone, borneol, camphene and cineol. It has been used as a choleretic for nearly 30 years and has recently been shown to lower the cholesterol saturation of bile. Preliminary reports indicate that it can dissolve stones in the gall bladder as well as in the common bile duct but experience is too limited to quote a success rate. The combination of Rowachol and a small dose of CDCA (375 mg/day) seems to be more effective than either alone and could be an attractive alternative to CDCA since it is substantially cheaper and seldom causes diarrhoea. Rowachol seems to be a safe preparation but its use in treating gall-stones must still be regarded as experimental.

Surgical Treatment of Gall-stones

Cholecystectomy is still the most appropriate treatment for most patients with gall-stones. In competent hands, elective removal of the gall bladder is as safe as an abdominal operation can be. Recurrence is, of course, impossible but there is a small risk of common duct stones being left behind, even after operative cholangiography. Cholecystectomy is followed by an increased incidence of cancer of the right colon, but the risk is still very small.

Complications of Gall-stones and Their Treatment

Acute Cholecystitis

This usually presents as an acute abdomen with right upper quadrant pain and tenderness, fever and leucocytosis. It is normally regarded as an absolute indication for surgery but there is dispute as to whether operation is best performed early or late. Most surgeons favour early but not immediate surgery. Immediate treatment consists of intravenous fluids, fasting, analgesics other than opiates and, in severe cases, antibiotics. Commonly used antibiotics are ampicillin or amoxycillin, cephalosporins and gentamicin. An extra reason for antibiotics is to reduce post-operative wound infection.

Stones in the Common Bile Duct (Choledocholithiasis)

Choledocholithiasis can be symptomless but usually presents with cholestatic jaundice. Sometimes this is associated with biliary-type pain and sometimes with the features of bacterial cholangitis including fever, tenderness in the right upper quadrant and leucocytosis. Unrelieved, choledocholithiasis can lead to irreversible liver damage (secondary biliary cirrhosis), hepatic abscesses or septicaemia. Therefore, in symptomatic cases, treatment is urgent and normally consists of surgical exploration of the common duct, often combined with choledochoduodenostomy.

In centres with special endoscopic expertise, stones can be let out of the duct by endoscopic sphincterotomy, with or without extraction, using a device such as the Dormier basket. This is significantly safer than re-operation but entails some risk of bleeding and septicaemia.

If a T-tube is still in situ when retained stones are discovered, three other options are available: (a) allow the T-tube track to "mature" for 4–6 weeks, then remove it and pass instruments down the track into the common duct to extract the stones; (b) flush the tube with saline to try and wash the stones out through the ampulla of Vater (this seldom succeeds) and (c) perfuse the tube with a solution designed to dissolve the stones in situ. Many solutions have been tried but only two have been well documented. A solution of 100 mM sodium cholate is moderately effective but causes severe diarrhoea. At present, mono-octanoin seems the material of choice. This is a medium chain monoglyceride with detergent properties and a good capacity to solubilise cholesterol. In one series 24 patients with ductal stones were infused with mono-octanoin at 2–4 ml/h. Complete dissolution occurred in 15 patients, usually within a week, and partial dissolution in another five. At this slow infusion rate diarrhoea was rare. Biliary pain occurred occasionally but subsided when bile was aspirated.

When there is no T-tube in place, the stones are radiolucent and not too large, and symptoms are mild or absent, it is worth trying oral CDCA or UDCA. These are successful in, at best, half the patients but the success rate may be improved by adding Rowachol. The main disadvantage of oral treatment is its slowness. Also, it is necessary to use intravenous cholangiography [or endoscopic retrograde cholangio-pancreatography (ERCP)] to monitor its effect.

Acute Pancreatitis

Many if not most attacks of acute pancreatitis are associated with the passage of a gall-stone into the intestine. One of the benefits of treating gall-stones is the avoidance of this feared complication. The management of acute pancreatitis is discussed in Chap. 9.

Acalculous Cholecystitis

This is an uncommon condition, accounting for only 2% of cases of acute cholecystitis. In some cases it is likely that stones were present but were passed at the time of the attack. In the rest, the pathogenesis is obscure. It can occur at the same time as another infection, especially in diabetics, in children with streptococcal infections, in patients with neoplastic disease and when there are congenital anomalies of the biliary or vascular systems. The clinical features are not distinctive, but the disease is more often severe than calculous cholecystitis. Treatment is the same but surgical mortality is higher.

Sclerosing Cholangitis

This is a rare, chronic, fibrosing, inflammatory process involving the larger bile ducts. About one-third of patients have ulcerative colitis. Other associations include retroperitoneal fibrosis, sclerosing mediastinitis, Riedel's thyroiditis and relapsing pancreatitis. It usually presents with jaundice, right hypochondrial discomfort, pruritus and occasional fever. Malaise and weight loss are common. Late complications are portal hypertension and liver cell failure.

Unfortunately, no treatment is known which alters the relentless progression of this disease. Corticosteroids, azathioprine and antibiotics have been tried without benefit. In severe cases, surgical intubation of the biliary system should be attempted, if only to relieve symptoms. As with any prolonged cholestasis, the fat-soluble vitamins should be given by monthly injection with regular calcium supplements. If steatorrhoea is severe, medium-chain triglycerides and a low fat diet may be helpful. Treatment of underlying colitis, even colectomy, seems to have little effect.

Further Reading

Bell GD (1979) Medical treatment of gallstones. J Roy Coll Physicians Lond 13: 47–52

Dowling RH (1977) Chenodeoxycholic acid therapy of gallstones. Clin Gastroenterol 6: 141–163

Dowling RH (1979) The gallstone dissolution story. Hosp Update 1081–1103

Ellis WR, Bell GD (1981) Treatment of biliary duct stones with a terpene preparation. Br Med J 282: 611

Ellis WR, Bell GD, Middleton B, White DA (1981) Adjunct to bile acid treatment for gallstone dissolution: low-dose chenodeoxycholic acid combined with a terpene preparation. Br Med J 282: 611–612

Jarrett WN, Balfour TW, Bell GD, Knapp DR, Rose DH (1981) Intraductal infusion of monooctanoin: experience in 24 patients with retained common-duct stones. Lancet I: 68–70

Maton PM, Murphy GM, Dowling RH (1977) Ursodeoxycholic acid treatment of gallstones. Dose-response study and possible mechanism of action. Lancet II: 1297–1301

Schoenfield LJ (1977) Diseases of the gallbladder and biliary system. Wiley, New York

Thistle JL, Hofmann AF, Otto BJ, Stephens DH (1978) Chenotherapy for gallstone dissolution. I. Efficacy and safety. JAMA 239: 1041–1046

8 Hepatic Disease
A. E. Read

Viral Hepatitis

Pathophysiology

Several viruses cause an acute generalised inflammation of the liver parenchyma, i.e. hepatitis. At the time of writing three viruses, A, B and a non-A non-B (which may exist in more than one form) are of greatest clinical importance. In epidemic form these diseases are easy to identify as they cause similar illnesses characterised by the fairly sudden onset of pyrexia, anorexia, nausea and vomiting, and later jaundice. Sporadic cases are more difficult to identify. *Virus A* is spread by oral–faecal contamination, and virus B and non-A non-B are commonly seen after blood transfusion or the use of contaminated syringes or instruments in susceptible people. In respect of virus B the importance of sexual transmission, particularly in the male homosexual, is now widely recognised, whilst non-A non-B infection may be more common in drug abusers.

Diagnosis in all types rests on the existence of a compatible history and clinical signs. Liver function tests show disordered hepatocellular function, and in the case of virus A and virus B infection there are appropriate diagnostic immunological tests on the blood.

Therapeutic Principles

The aim is to support liver function whilst awaiting the resolution of the disease. The average case is best treated with bed rest, at least until the fever has settled. The patient can be allowed up to toilet as at the stage at which he is symptomatic; the stools of virus A patients are not infective. Nausea and anorexia are combated by providing a light nutritious diet containing a minimum of fat, with plenty of glucose-containing drinks. Treatment can usually be continued without hospital admission. It is important to establish early on whether the patient is hepatitis B positive or not, as this affects the long-term and immediate prognosis and also means that very strict precautions must be taken in dealing with blood and other body fluids in virus B positive cases.

Liver function is supported by ensuring adequate caloric intake. Bed rest is essential where jaundice is moderately severe and where fever and constitutional symptoms persist. The dangers and pitfalls are firstly the failure to differentiate viral hepatitis from other types of hepatic jaundice such as that due to drugs and alcohol, and secondly to confuse it with primary obstructive disease of the biliary tree, either at an intra- or extra-hepatic level. Nor must the warning signs of progression of acute hepatitis to acute hepatic necrosis or to chronic hepatitis be missed. In the former, deepening jaundice, a haemorrhagic tendency, delirium and renal shut-down accompany a reduction in hepatic size, whilst in the latter persistent jaundice, increasing splenomegaly, fluid retention and the appearance of cutaneous signs of chronic liver disease, e.g. spider naevi, are possible clues.

Drug Treatment

Corticosteroids

Corticosteroids have been widely used, particularly in moderately severe and severe cases of hepatitis, or where activity of the disease is prolonged (e.g. jaundice >1 month). It is well recognised, however, that the use of corticosteroid drugs is fraught with some hazards. Firstly, because of impaired liver cell function there is impaired metabolism of corticosteroids, and treatment is therefore associated with an increased incidence of side-effects such as weight gain and psychosis. Secondly, their local ulcerative effect on the gastric mucosa, perhaps in the presence of prolonged blood coagulation caused by impaired hepatic synthesis of coagulant factors, may lead to troublesome gastrointestinal bleeding. However, in severe cases of hepatitis corticosteroids given orally, 30 mg prednisolone daily in divided doses, are usually effective in producing (a) a non-specific increase in well-being and appetite and (b) a decrease in the patient's jaundice and a commensurate fall in the serum bilirubin value.

Treatment with corticosteroids should be continued in decreasing doses until the serum bilirubin value is normal and until the rest of the liver function tests show a significant improvement. A too rapid cessation of treatment may sometimes be associated with a relapse in which the clinical and biochemical status is as bad or worse than in the original attack.

The mode of action of corticosteroids in acute hepatitis is uncertain. On the one hand cynics have suggested that the major effect is one of bilirubin disposal, and that no beneficial effect on the basic disease is seen—certainly the histological damage seems not to be affected. On the other hand the rapid improvement in other parameters of liver function and the fact that in some forms of chronic liver cell disease a beneficial effect of corticosteroids on hepatic protein synthesis has been demonstrated, makes some beneficial effect on the disease process likely.

A recent trial of corticosteroids in Dallas, Texas showed no advantage in the corticosteroid group. Certainly care is needed in the selection of patients who require this treatment.

Cyanidamol (Catechin)

Cyanidamol is a bioflavin and has been shown to have a number of actions which could be beneficial to the damaged liver cell. These include increasing the NADH/NAD ratio, raising levels of adenosine triphosphate and stabilising lysosomal membranes. In a hundred patients with acute viral hepatitis the disappearance of HBsAg from the blood was accelerated in virus B cases, and there was a more rapid disappearance of symptoms and fall of the serum bilirubin compared with controls. The trial was a double-blind one. The drug is given in a dose of 2 g daily. The precise place of this substance in the treatment of acute hepatitis is uncertain.

Drugs to Be Avoided

In general it may be expected that acute hepatitis may accentuate the effects of many drugs simply because of the resultant impairment of hepatic metabolism. All drugs must therefore be used with caution, and if required, are given at reduced dosage in affected patients. Further, it is of course unwise to use drugs which are capable of producing hepatotoxicity, even if this is a rare hypersensitivity phenomenon (see p. 130). Drugs which accentuate the features of liver cell failure such as sedatives, sodium and fluid-retaining compounds, and drugs which may cause gastric irritation and ulceration with possible resultant bleeding are also to be avoided.

Complications

The major complications of the disease are:

1. Progression to acute hepatic necrosis—this has a high mortality (>80%)

2. Progression to chronic liver disease and eventually to cirrhosis (not in virus A cases)

3. Acute aplastic anaemia and polyarteritis nodosa; these are occasional serious complications, the latter being confined to virus B hepatitis

4. A troublesome but benign disorder, "the posthepatitis syndrome"; this is common, and because it is associated with continuing ill health, anorexia, fatigue and dyspepsia cause a high morbidity. The disorder is probably psychogenic, though like many other viral illnesses, hepatitis may be a genuine cause of marked postinfective debility.

Acute Hepatic Necrosis

Principles of Management

Acute hepatic necrosis is a difficult condition to treat, and the multitude of treatments available is evidence of the extremely unsatisfactory results of therapy. Corticosteroid drugs are not only thought to be unhelpful, but frankly dangerous, and they are not recommended.

The patient is kept on a full antihepatic coma regime (see p. 126) of no oral feeding of protein, neomycin to sterilise the large bowel and i.v. strong glucose solutions by a central venous catheter. Careful monitoring of the serum potassium is carried out, as both dangerous hypokalaemia and hyperkalaemia —the latter in association with renal failure, when it is almost always fatal— may occur.

Apart from supportive treatment, haemodialysis, exchange transfusion and perfusion through an isolated or intact human or animal liver have all been unsuccessful. Slightly more success has been reported using perfusion of the patient's blood through a silicone-coated charcoal column, and the use of dialysis using polyacrylonitrile membranes is under trial at the moment. These two latter techniques have been performed in one specialist unit where a very high standard of intensive patient care may explain any improvement in mortality obtained.

Great care must be taken to avoid any sedative and sodium-retaining agents in this condition and to monitor and treat where possible hypoglycaemia or any haemorrhagic condition that develops.

Chronic Active Hepatitis

Pathophysiology

This is a chronic generalised inflammatory disease of the liver which progresses to cirrhosis. A number of causes are recognised, including:

1. An autoimmune variety due to cell-mediated immunological damage to the liver, most commonly seen in women. The $HLAB_8$ and DW_3 antigens are more frequently found in sufferers than in controls, and multi-organ involvement is common

2. Due to persisting infection with hepatitis B or non-A non-B virus

3. As a result of liver damage with drugs such as methyldopa, oxyphenisatin, isoniazid, dantrolene sodium and perhexiline maleate

4. Idiopathic, due to unknown causes. (The part played by, for example, the virus of non-A non-B hepatitis in this group is uncertain.)

Therapeutic Principles

The aim of therapy is to suppress the activity of the inflammatory process in the liver and thus hopefully to prevent the progression to cirrhosis. In effect, although good evidence of improvement of liver cell function and lessening of inflammatory processes in the liver is seen following therapy, cirrhosis, which is often present at an early stage, is not prevented. For this reason successful medical treatment, though lessening the activity of liver cell disease, leaves the patient with the mechanical (e.g. portal hypertension) and other problems of a cirrhotic liver.

Non-drug Management

This is very important where there is possibly a drug cause of the disease. These cases must be clearly identified by careful history taking and ever present vigilance in the detection of drug-induced liver disease, because of the gratifying response that many show to cessation of the offending drug.

Drug Treatment

Corticosteroids

A beneficial effect of corticosteroids is to be expected in this disease, and most particularly where an immunological aetiology is likely. Treatment results in suppression of evidence of activity of the disease, i.e. a fall in serum bilirubin values, a fall in transaminases and serum globulins and a rise in the serum albumin. Clinically, apart from the lessening of jaundice, the patient feels better, and where there is evidence of multi-organ involvement this is often improved too. Thus skin rashes, arthralgia, haemolytic anaemia and the symptoms and signs of ulcerative colitis may all improve. Histologically, there is evidence of improvement of liver cell damage, but the progression to cirrhosis (if this is not already present) is not halted.

Corticosteroids may have significant side-effects in patients with chronic liver disease, related to their slower rate of hepatic metabolism. Thus mooning, striae and even serious complications such as psychosis may occur, so that corticosteroids must not be used unless the diagnosis is correct. Further variable binding of corticosteroids by a changing serum albumin level may mean that drug dosage has to be altered to obtain the required therapeutic effect. Treatment is usually begun with prednisone or prednisolone (most workers feel that there is no great advantage in using the latter), and initial high doses are tailed off to a maintenance dose of 5–15 mg daily. A careful watch must be kept for side-effects, remembering that patients are often young and female, and extremely conscious of their appearance. In this respect azathioprine is a useful steroid-sparing agent. Therapy is continued until liver function tests are normal. A gradual withdrawal of treatment is then possible, though relapse which needs further treatment occurs in about 60% of patients. Eventually with time and treatment it may be possible to keep the patient off steroids permanently, though he or she is invariably cirrhotic at this stage.

Azathioprine (Imuran)

This drug is metabolised in the liver to 6-mercaptopurine. It is inferior to corticosteroids in the treatment of this disease and is certainly never used as an initial or only treatment. Not only is there little evidence of improvement with this drug alone, but occasionally a serious deterioration in liver function takes place. Azathioprine is valuable, however, in combination with corticosteroids, with which it seems to act synergistically. It allows a reduction of the dose of corticosteroid required to control the disease. A small dose of azathioprine, e.g. 50 mg daily, is usually used, and complications are unusual though routine haematological monitoring is a wise precaution.

The maintenance dose of azathioprine and prednisolone required for treatment of this condition is thus usually 50 mg azathioprine and 10 mg prednisolone.

Hepatitis B Positive Chronic Active Hepatitis

The treatment of this form of chronic active hepatitis presents difficulties. It is generally thought, for example, that virus B cases respond poorly to treatment with immunosuppressant drugs, and there is evidence to suggest that their use might allow the virus to replicate, perhaps because of diminished immune function. Most clinicians faced with the problem of chronic active hepatitis due to virus B would therefore consider the implications very carefully before giving immunosuppressive drugs. There is reason to believe that virus B cases are generally milder and have little tendency to multi-organ involvement. Further, such cases are rare in this country. If, however, such a case presents and activity is associated with symptoms and deteriorating liver cell function, a trial of corticosteroids with azathioprine is worthwhile. A search for other agents which may be effective in this condition has led to trials of (a) high titre specific immune anti-HB_s, (b) levamisole and transfer factor (which stimulate the immune system), (c) interferon and (d) adenine arabinoside 5'mono-phosphate (ARA-AMP). Success has been claimed for the last two in this list, but availability and expense are obviously serious limiting factors, and the results are not particularly impressive.

Drugs to Be Avoided

Care must be taken with any drugs which are likely to produce fluid retention, cause sedation or possibly lead to gastric irritation and intestinal haemorrhage.

Most drugs, including prednisolone, are more slowly metabolised in patients with this type of liver disease, and reduced dosage and careful clinical monitoring are required.

Complications

The complications of chronic active hepatitis are:

1. Progression to hepatic cirrhosis, whether or not the patient is treated — this course is usual.

2. Liver cell failure, which is an integral part of the disease. It may be exacerbated by intercurrent infection or by an alimentary bleed. This feature of the disease is often controlled by immunosuppressive therapy.

3. Multiple autoimmune disorders, which are a feature of the immunological variety of the disease.

4. Hepatoma—though rare, this becomes a more important problem with long-term survival.

Prognosis

About 40% of patients with chronic active hepatitis die within 5 years of presentation. Death is usually due to liver cell failure; less often it is due to sepsis or other related immunological disorders. Survival with an inactive cirrhosis still renders the patient susceptible to conditions like portal hypertension, and with time liver cell function deteriorates and the features of chronic liver cell failure may be seen.

Primary Biliary Cirrhosis

Pathophysiology

This is a chronic disease of the liver based on an intrahepatic obstruction of the biliary tree at the level of the small bile ducts. This process is caused by an immunologically mediated mechanism; eventually a fine micronodular cirrhosis results. The disease is one of middle age and is strikingly more common in women. Though most patients have symptoms due to obstructive jaundice, i.e. icterus with pale stools and dark urine and pruritus, many patients may be asymptomatic and special tests may be required, either serological or biochemical, to make the diagnosis.

Therapeutic Principles

These are fourfold:

1. As the patient has chronic obstructive jaundice, it is essential to prevent deficiencies of the fat-soluble vitamins, particularly vitamins A, D and K. Serious complications may occur if this is not done.

2. Pruritus, which may be a most distressing complication of the disease, must be controlled.

3. Liver cell failure and portal hypertension are usually but not always late manifestations of the disease. These may require urgent medical and surgical treatment.

4. It seems possible that treatments aimed at either the primary immunological problem or the secondary metabolic consequences, e.g. copper deposition, will become more effective and may be worthy of trial.

Non-drug Treatment

The judicious use of make-up in females is an important psychological prop, as darkening of the skin may lead to concern and embarrassment. Similarly, a low-fat diet may help to reduce the severity of diarrhoea.

Drug Treatment

Treatment of Vitamin Deficiency

Prophylactic vitamin supplements are required for all patients with primary biliary cirrhosis, and certainly prophylactic vitamin K is required to prevent excessive bleeding and vitamin D to prevent tetany and bone disease. These vitamins are conveniently given by i.m. injection as vitamin K 10–20 mg and vitamin D 50 000 units each month. In the face of deficiency causing clinical symptoms these doses need to be increased, as may the dose of vitamin K prior to even minor surgery such as tooth extraction. Some patients with bone disease (osteomalacia) may in fact be refractory to vitamin D_3 (calciferol) given by injection. The newer vitamin D analogues such as one-alpha (1α-OH vitamin D_3), which is rapidly converted in the liver to 1,25-dihydroxy-vitamin D_3, may then be useful. Use of this drug requires biochemical monitoring of serum calcium, and it is given orally, initially in a dose of 1 μg and then at a maintenance dose of 0.25–1 μg/day. Suspicion of the presence of vitamin A deficiency, e.g. from impaired night vision or dry skin, would be an indicator for supplements of this vitamin too (e.g. vitamin A tablets, 50 000 units, one tablet daily for 10 days). The use of cholestyramine (see below) would be a further warning as to the need for vitamin D and K therapy.

Pruritus

Simple sedative skin lotions, such as calamine lotion with 1% phenol, or the use of a *small* dose of an antihistamine may be all that is required. In those patients in whom pruritus is a severe problem, cholestyramine, a bile salt binding agent, may be useful. This agent given by mouth binds intraluminal bile salts, which then bypass the ileal absorptive site and are excreted in the faeces. This leads to a reduction of the bile salt pool and subsequently a decrease in the elevated serum and tissue bile salt levels. Pruritus, which is somehow mediated by bile salts fixed in the skin, is relieved. By reducing luminal bile salt levels in the gut, cholestyramine is likely to exacerbate steatorrhoea and may interfere with the absorption of a variety of drugs, and particularly the fat-soluble vitamins.

Cholestyramine is given as an orange-flavoured powder (Questran) one to three sachets (9–27 g) daily. Each sachet supplies 4 g of anhydrous cholestyramine. Unflavoured it is unpleasant to take, and compliance is not high unless severe pruritus is significantly relieved. Relief does not occur if biliary obstruction is complete because of the inability of cholestyramine and bile salts to bind in the gut.

Other bile salt binding agents such as Aludrox may also be effective in treating pruritus, as may be the use of ultraviolet light.

Preservation of Liver Cell Function

It is difficult to preserve liver cell function, but infection and alimentary bleeding must be effectively treated. Not only may the patient bleed—usually late in the disease from oesophageal varices complicating portal hypertension —but there is also an increased incidence of peptic ulcer and consequent haemorrhage. Cimetidine is useful in patients with proven peptic ulcer, in whom it should be given as long-term prophylaxis. Should it be shown that alimentary bleeding is due to erosive gastritis—a not uncommon event in chronic liver disease—treatment in the acute phase with cimetidine and regular oral antacids may also be helpful, though evidence concerning this is conflicting.

Bleeding associated with portal hypertension may require medical or surgical treatment, e.g. sclerosis of varices or even a shunt operation. Deeply jaundiced patients, however, tolerate such surgical procedures poorly: vitamin K by injection and adequate hydration are important preliminaries to surgery.

Treatment of the Disease Process

There is nothing that can be done to reverse the obliterative process in the biliary tree. Trials of corticosteroids and azathioprine have largely been unsuccessful. Further, there are important reasons (see below) for avoiding corticosteroids. Penicillamine has immunosuppressive properties and might therefore be of use in this disease. In addition to this, D-penicillamine is known to be an effective copper chelating agent, and it is widely recognised that copper—which is normally excreted in the bile—is retained within the liver in cholestasis, where it could possibly produce secondary hepatic damage. Actually this factor is probably overemphasised, and it must of course be remembered that penicillamine has a number of important side-effects. These include blood dyscrasias, proteinuria, skin rashes, myasthenia and a drug-induced lupus syndrome. Great care must therefore be taken, and penicillamine is probably not effective in all cases. On doses of 600 mg to 1 g a day, an improvement of liver function tests and histological improvement can be found, but side-effects are often prohibitive. A low dose regime, e.g. 250 mg daily, may also be helpful without having serious side-effects. Regular clinical monitoring, examination of urine and measurement of blood count are essential if this drug is used. Modern opinion suggests perhaps paradoxically that penicillamine therapy should be reserved for symptomatic rather than mild cases. The latter often have a good prognosis even when untreated. A recent study from the Royal Free Hospital shows an improved mortality in late-stage disease with penicillamine.

Drugs to Be Avoided

The usual warnings concerning the dangers of sedative drugs (including antihistamines given for pruritus) to patients with liver disease are important here. Drugs which cause fluid retention or which might exacerbate hepatic encephalopathy must be used sparingly. Corticosteroids are contra-indicated. Biliary obstruction in this disease is not improved by their use, and they may worsen osteoporosis, encourage the appearance of peptic ulceration (perhaps with gastrointestinal bleeding) and cause a rapid increase in weight and severe corticosteroid side-effects related to impaired drug metabolism.

Complications

The complications of this disease include portal hypertension with bleeding from oesophageal varices, and liver cell failure. These either alone or in combination are the ultimate cause of death. In cases of usual severity this occurs about 5 years after presentation. There are exceptions to this rule, and mild cases (without significant jaundice) may fare much better.

Wilson's Disease

Pathophysiology

This is a congenital disorder inherited as an autosomal recessive trait. It is associated with abnormally high levels of copper in various tissues in the body, but in particular in the liver, kidneys and brain. Conversely, serum concentrations of copper are low. Tissue damage results in the liver (hepatic cirrhosis), brain (degeneration in basal ganglia) and kidney (renal tubular damage) etc.

Drug Treatment

Identification of this disease is extremely important as this is one of the forms of chronic liver disease which significantly benefits from specific treatment, though the cirrhosis is probably irreversible. The identification of this disease is an absolute indication for the use of D-penicillamine. In the rare cases where the side-effects of D-penicillamine are such that treatment is impossible, Trilene is an alternative. D-Penicillamine is commenced as 1.2 g in four divided doses daily before meals. Urinary copper excretion is measured to make sure that urinary copper-loss is increased. Up to 3 g/day can be given; this seriously increases the risk of serious side-effects, but these are less common in Wilson's disease than in other situations. Most patients are maintained on a dose of 1–1.5 g/day. In the initial stages there may well be an intensification of neurological features, and in any case progress may be very slow. Mental function and handwriting are good tests of progress. Treatment may be required for 1–2 years before evidence of improvement is obtained, and the dose of D-penicillamine may have to be increased. Treatment is a life sentence. Non-responsive cases may be considered for hepatic transplantation.

Alcoholic Liver Disease

Pathophysiology

In susceptible patients alcohol in sufficient quantities (usually >80 g/day) will produce a variety of hepatic pathological changes from mild and reversible fatty infiltration to complete and irreversible cirrhosis. The precise cause of these changes is not known, and no doubt in some the effect is a direct toxic one on the hepatocytes, whilst in others genetic predisposition and dietary and immunological factors may all be important. Alcoholic cirrhosis is, for example, more common in England in patients wth $HLAB_8$ than it should be.

Therapeutic Principles

The important function of the physician is to encourage the patient to abstain permanently from alcohol. This may be realised by ancillary drug therapy or with the help of family, friends, a psychiatrist and organisations such as Alcoholics Anonymous.

The complications of alcoholic liver disease are:

1. Neurological
    a) Cerebral: delirium tremens, Korsakoff's psychosis
    b) Brain stem: central myelinolysis, Wernicke's encephalopathy
    c) Peripheral nerves: peripheral neuropathy
2. Haematological: bone marrow suppression, haemolytic anaemia, megaloblastic anaemia
3. Muscular: acute myopathy
4. Gastrointestinal: pancreatitis, gastritis, peptic ulcer, diarrhoea
5. Nutritional: vitamin deficiency (particularly vitamin B)

The treatment of all the above complications revolves around the elimination of alcohol intake and the correction of nutritional deficiencies.

The diagnosis of alcoholic liver disease may be very difficult—not all patients will admit to excessive intake, and some will have little evidence of liver disease or will present with evidence of organ dysfunction outside the liver, e.g. peripheral neuropathy. Alternatively some types of severe liver disease may mimic closely a variety of non-alcoholic hepatic disorders. Careful clinical observation is supplemented by questioning of the patients and his or her family and friends and, of course, by diagnostic—particularly histological—tests.

Non-drug Management

Abstinence from alcohol is essential and anything that can be done to achieve this end is important. Thus changing jobs from one with a risk, e.g. a publican or entertainer, to one where the risk is less may help, as may the settling of financial or personal problems or the treatment of psychiatric illness such as depression. Hospital admission, heavy sedation and aversion therapy with drugs such as disulfiram may all be helpful in individual cases.

Nutritional deficiencies must be protected against by encouraging a full diet with a liberal protein intake except, that is, where hepatic encephalopathy is suspected. Where wasting and anorexia are problems, enteric feeding through a small bore nasal tube may be very helpful. Vitamin B supplements are essential, particularly where there is peripheral neuropathy or Wernicke's encephalopathy.

Drug Treatment of Alcohol Withdrawal

The danger of alcohol withdrawal is the onset of alarming neurological complications—delirium tremens—with a not insignificant mortality. Chlormethiazole (Heminevrin) by slow i.v. infusion 300–800 mg (0.8% sol. at about 60 drops/min) via a drip, or oral chlordiazepoxide 15–200 mg daily or chlorpromazine 25–50 mg three times daily is given to prevent such complications.

Drug Treatment of Alcoholic Liver Disease

No specific therapy is available, and indeed in the less severe forms of alcoholic liver disease none is necessary. Patient well-being, biochemistry and histology improve with withdrawal of alcohol and treatment with a hospital diet supplemented with large doses of vitamins.

In cases where there is evidence of deep jaundice and other aspects of liver cell failure, the lack of effective therapy is a serious deficiency. These patients are often pyrexial with massive hepatomegaly and evidence on liver biopsy of gross liver cell damage and spotty areas of necrosis. This is usually called acute alcoholic hepatitis and an underlying cirrhosis may or may not be present as well. Various forms of therapy have been tried.

Corticosteroids

In view of the fact that the clinical picture in alcoholic hepatitis is not unlike that of chronic active hepatitis, it seemed reasonable to try corticosteroids in these ill patients. Many trials have in fact been performed, and there seems to be no conclusive evidence that these agents are helpful. In very severe cases where there is real concern as to the patient's ability to survive and where deep jaundice and features such as ascites and prolongation of coagulation studies are present, a trial of prednisolone 40 mg daily may well be worthwhile. Against this possible benefit must be placed the real hazards of encouraging infection, gastrointestinal haemorrhage and hypokalaemia.

Propylthiouracil

Following the experimental recognition of the centrilobular distribution of alcohol-induced liver disease in animals, its worsening by anoxia and its amelioration by thyroidectomy, it was suggested that the centrilobular damage due to alcohol was partially related to the induction by alcohol of a hypermetabolic state and subsequent development of centrilobular tissue anoxia. This led to the trial of propylthiouracil by Orrego and colleagues from Toronto in patients with alcoholic liver disease. Clinical and biochemical evidence of alcohol-induced liver disease was more rapidly controlled by propylthiouracil 300 mg/day than by a placebo. This was seen in those with severe (alcoholic hepatitis and cirrhosis) rather than mild (fatty liver and inactive cirrhosis) cases. Propylthiouracil is certainly worth trying in the very worrying patient with severe liver disease of alcoholic aetiology not responding to intensive feeding and conservative therapy.

Hepatic Vein Thrombosis

Pathophysiology

This serious hepatic disorder has many causes. Basically these differ depending on whether occlusion is of the small centrilobular veins within the liver or of the major hepatic veins e.g. by thrombosis in polycythaemia vera.[1] In the former case, the cause may be veno-occlusive disease or drugs such as alcohol (central hyaline sclerosis); in the latter, thrombosis may result from (a) trauma, (b) underlying blood disease associated with clotting, e.g. polycythaemia, paroxysmal nocturnal haemoglobinuria, (c) drugs causing clotting, e.g. the pill, (d) tumours invading hepatic veins, e.g. renal carcinoma and hepatoma, and (e) congenital vena caval webs.

[1] A similar picture but without hepatic vein occlusion is associated with a chronically raised right atrial pressure, e.g. due to constrictive pericarditis.

The result of hepatic venous occlusion is intense centrilobular congestion of the liver, with necrosis and focal haemorrhage. The liver swells and the intrasinusoidal and portal capillary pressure increases. Local exudation of lymph from the surface of the liver and the portal circulation causes ascites. Patients who survive the disease may develop pseudolobulation and a true hepatic cirrhosis.

Therapeutic Principles

The aim of treatment is to support liver function so that the remaining surviving liver tissue has time to compensate for the acute liver cell failure. Treatment of ascites is also important, and in those who survive the initial onslaught and enter a subacute phase attention must be directed to the possibility of providing effective venous drainage from the liver by portocaval anastomosis. Most important of all, underlying conditions such as polycythaemia vera or (rarely) "congenital" webs across the inferior vena cava need early detection and treatment.

Drug Treatment

Anticoagulants

Although theoretically administration of anticoagulants would appear to be an entirely sensible form of therapy in order to prevent extension of thrombosis, a haemorrhagic disorder caused by the onset of liver cell failure is soon seen in many patients. It is then inappropriate to add anticoagulants to an already dangerous situation. In rare cases where this order of events is not seen, anticoagulants may be used. They are obviously particularly important when primary disorders of coagulation such as polycythaemia are present, and in follow-up treatment.

Diuretics

Diuretics are given in full dosage, as previously documented. Diuretics may, however, be only partially successful and rapidly accumulating ascites may have to be tapped. Diuretics are in any case potentially dangerous in patients with liver cell failure (see p. 126), and electrolyte disturbances and impaired renal perfusion may readily result.

Non-drug Management

Diet

Intense fluid accumulation in the abdomen and a failure of diuretic therapy to control this would be an indication for dietary restriction of sodium intake.

Progressive liver failure would also be an indication for reducing protein in the diet or eliminating it altogether.

Surgery

In patients who survive the onset of hepatic venous thrombosis and in whom the diagnosis is confirmed by investigations such as liver biopsy (if coagulation studies permit), technetium scanning and inferior vena cavography, the possibility of providing effective venous drainage from the liver by side-to-side portocaval anastamosis or more simply by a Dacron H graft between the portal vein or superior mesenteric vein and inferior vena cava must be considered. In fact, it may be impossible to contemplate surgery in patients deteriorating from progressive liver failure, but in those who stabilise such an operation may allow improvement, loss of ascites and an opportunity for liver cell function to improve.

Other Therapy

In those patients found to have hepatic venous thrombosis secondary to polycythaemia, urgent treatment—firsty by venesection supplemented by anticoagulants, and secondly by the use of radioactive phosphorus therapy or busulphan—must be given.

Drugs to Be Avoided

These are as outlined for other disorders in which chronic liver cell dysfunction occurs.

Liver Cell Failure

Pathophysiology

In any condition in which generalised liver damage occurs, the syndrome of liver cell failure may be seen. The disorder may occur acutely in patients with previously normal livers if a generalised disease such as viral hepatitis or a drug hepatitis affects the liver, or more chronically in patients with hepatic disorders such as cirrhosis. Patients with cirrhosis may remain relatively well and have few or none of the clinical features of the syndrome. Then some acute metabolic insult such as that resulting from intercurrent infection or an alimentary bleed makes the syndrome clinically obvious.

The syndrome of liver cell failure is characterised clinically by:

1. *Jaundice* due basically to impaired liver cell metabolism of bilirubin and diminished biliary flow secondary to bile salt deficiency. Note that in some cirrhotics cholestasis may be a further cause of jaundice, for which gall-stones or hepatoma may be responsible.

2. *Fluid retention*, which is due basically to impaired renal handling of sodium augmented by increased transfer of fluid into the tissues associated with hypoalbuminaemia, and the "weeping" of hepatic lymph into the abdominal cavity.

3. *Hepatic encephalopathy*, of which the precise cause is uncertain but which probably represents the effects of intoxication of deep centres in the brain whose activity is normally associated with awareness. A variety of neurological syndromes may be produced.

4. *A bleeding diathesis*, which may be due to a variety of causes but is most usually the result of deficient production of coagulant factors in the liver and the sequestration of platelets in the spleen (thrombocytopenia) and platelet dysfunction.

Therapeutic Principles

The aim of treatment is to support the liver and preserve such function as it has whilst avoiding situations which could further compromise it.

It is important to distinguish between liver cell failure in those whose liver function was previously normal and in those in whom liver cell failure is a manifestation of underlying chronic liver disease—the prognosis is significantly different.

Non-drug Management

Patients must be treated with bed rest. All sedative, analgesic and neuroleptic drugs are contra-indicated.

Diet must be nutritious, and in view of the almost invariable presence of clinical or latent hepatic encephalopathy a low protein diet 40 g/24 h (or less) and full vitamin supplements are required. Sodium containing drugs or i.v. infusions are contra-indicated, as are drugs with a known fluid-retaining effect. Great care must be taken to ensure that infections—including bloodstream infection—are rapidly diagnosed and treated. Diabetes is not uncommon in patients with chronic liver disease, and its effective treatment may bring about a considerable improvement in nutritional status. Provision of adequate nutrition remains an important problem in patients with chronic liver cell disease. Hepatic encephalopathy prevents adequate provision of nutrition despite the considerable evidence of wasting and malnutrition that can be present, and anorexia is not helped by the use of low sodium-containing diets.

Acute Liver Cell Failure

In acute liver cell failure the treatment is purely supportive and the mortality is high. Apart from special centres which carry out perfusion of blood through columns of coated activated charcoal or haemodialysis using polyacrylonitrile membranes, there is no other treatment that will help. The mortality is of the order of 80%. Those who are elderly, who develop renal failure or who have a bleeding tendency are particularly likely to die.

Chronic Liver Cell Failure

Here it is extremely important to look for and energetically treat any precipitating event such as infection, intestinal bleeding or the injudicious use of sedative, analgesic, antidepressive or diuretic drugs. Complicating renal failure is also a common precipitant. Infection may be found in the lung or urinary tract, but it is particularly likely in the chest, ascitic fluid or bloodstream.

Drug Treatment

Jaundice

No drug is available that will reduce the serum bilirubin in patients with liver cell failure. Despite an early vogue for the use of corticosteroids (see below), it is now recognised that these agents can be dangerous, and their use except in certain special circumstances is contra-indicated.

Fluid Retention

Fluid retention should be carefully treated. Dietary sodium restriction is invariably required. Weight loss due to diuresis should be kept to 0.5 kg/day. Too rapid a diuresis may well contract the blood volume and decrease renal, hepatic and cerebral perfusion. Potassium-retaining diuretics are to be preferred, e.g. spironolactone 100–200 mg three times daily, but a careful watch must be kept on the serum potassium level. If loop or thiazide diuretics have to be given, potassium supplements are invariably required. Serum and urinary electrolytes must be monitored daily—a major disturbance of serum electrolytes is to be expected in 75% of patients; hyponatraemia is a particularly ominous sign. If ascites is present and causes distress, a small amount, e.g. a litre, may be removed to make the patient more comfortable.

Hepatic Encephalopathy

Dietary protein is carefully excluded, and a non-absorbable broad spectrum antibiotic such as neomycin 1 g three times daily is given by mouth. Ototoxicity may occur due to absorbed neomycin, particularly if renal function is poor (which is not unusual). Bowel movements are encouraged by saline purgatives such as magnesium sulphate supplemented by twice daily large bowel wash-outs.

Metronidazole is also a satisfactory antibiotic to give, and it is possible that neomycin and metronidazole act synergistically, on aerobes and anaerobes respectively.

Lactulose, a synthetic non-absorbable sugar, produces diarrhoea by exerting an osmotic effect in the bowel and is given by mouth 10–30 ml three times daily. In the gut, bacteria produce lactic and other organic acids from lactulose, the intestinal pH falls and the production of ammonia from gut bacterial activity diminishes. In some patients L-dopa and bromocriptine may also prove beneficial, presumably by encouraging the repletion of dopamine levels in the brain.

Bleeding Diathesis

Multiple causes may exist for a bleeding diathesis, which commonly complicates liver cell failure. The principal cause of the disorder is impaired hepatic synthesis of coagulant factors. For this reason therapy is usually difficult. Intramuscular vitamin K therapy may be helpful, but this is the exception rather than the rule because of underlying liver cell disease. Intravenous infusion of platelets may be helpful if patients have thrombocytopenia sufficient to cause spontaneous bleeding. Factor V deficiency may respond to infusion of intravenous fresh-frozen plasma. Agents which are liable to cause bleeding when taken orally, e.g. corticosteroids, must be rigorously excluded.

Summary

Though therapy of the sort outlined above may be helpful in controlling some of the manifestations of liver cell failure, the liver's capabilities of recovery are, unless it has been subject to an acute and reversible insult, limited. Replacement of the liver by transplantation is a possibility in those with underlying chronic liver disease, but this procedure is a major one, particularly in the compromised patient with liver failure, and a 1-year survival is to be expected in only about 20%. Cerebral oedema is an important finding contributing to death in some patients, particularly those with acute liver cell necrosis, and it is possible that i.v. mannitol or corticosteroids (best given by i.m. injection) may then be helpful.

Other therapeutic procedures include:

1. Haemoperfusion of the patient's blood through columns of coated charcoal granules (usually limited to cases of acute liver cell failure)

2. Haemodialysis using polyacrylonitrile membranes (limited to acute liver cell failure)

3. Exclusion of the colon by ileorectal anastomosis etc.—useful if chronic hepatic encephalopathy fails to respond to conservative treatment

4. Trials of classical haemodialysis, exchange transfusion, perfusion of the patient's blood through an isolated animal liver etc.—these have not been found to be helpful.

Hepatoma

Pathophysiology

These malignant tumours arise from the hepatocytes (liver cell carcinoma) or from the bile duct epithelium (cholangiocarcinoma). The former are by far the commonest and may occur either in a normal or in a cirrhotic liver. This is of great importance when considering the possibility of curative (surgical) therapy. The cause of the transformation of a cirrhotic liver into one where *multiple* foci of hepatoma are found is unknown. Hepatitis B virus may be implicated either as a direct cause of the tumour or of the underlying cirrhosis. Certain toxins, e.g. aflatoxin produced from moulds which may contaminate stored cereal grains, are known to be carcinogenic and could be important where hepatoma reaches almost epidemic proportions, such as tropical Africa. Drugs and hormones may have a part to play, and in respect to the latter the marked predominance of the tumour in males and the association between the administration of androgenic steroids and liver tumours is well appreciated. Less frequently, and particularly in the young, hepatoma—often a single massive lesion—is found in a normal liver.

Non-drug Treatment

Surgery may be curative in patients whose growth is solitary and where the underlying liver is normal. Laparoscopy and/or hepatic arteriography are used to assess the size and situation of the tumour. Formal right or left hepatic lobectomy, still a fairly major surgical procedure, allows complete eradication of the tumour providing it has not extended into the opposite lobe.

For those tumours which are multicentric and which complicate cirrhosis, only palliative treatment is usually possible, though hepatic transplantation is sometimes a possibility despite the tendency for secondary tumour spread outside the liver to then become clinically obvious. Attempts at palliation using hepatic artery ligation in order to shrink the tumour and to relieve pain have been partially successful but seem not to prolong life.

Drug Treatment

No antimitotic drug or combination of drugs is particularly helpful. Actinomycin (doxorubicin) does produce some evidence of remission in about one-third of patients treated. A dosage of 60 mg/m^2 at 3-weekly intervals reduces the distressing side-effects associated with administration over two or three successive days. Administration is via a freely running drip, 2–3 min being allowed to complete the injection. The cumulative dose of 550 mg/m^2 should only be exceeded if there is a good response. The dangers include congestive cardiac failure due to cardiomyopathy, bone marrow depression, alopecia, nausea and vomiting. The local risk of thrombophlebitis is minimised as indicated above. In the face of evidence of severe hepatocellular disease the dosage of this drug may have to be reduced by 50% or more.

Drug-Induced Liver Disease

Pathophysiology

A large number of drugs produce damage to the liver, either associated with damage to many organs, e.g. bone marrow and skin, or as a solitary phenomenon. Two major patterns of damage are found—*cholestasis* when there is evidence of biliary obstruction producing jaundice with pruritus, and *hepatocellular* when liver cell jaundice accompanies variable evidence of damage to other hepatic functions. These two major varieties are further subdivided and it must be remembered that a variety of less important hepatic disorders may be related to the taking of drugs. Little is known about mechanisms, but simple cholestasis may well represent the effects of disruption of bile salt absorption and excretion into the biliary canaliculus, and hence a failure of bile salt induced biliary flow. Interruption could be due to blockage of hepatic uptake, damage to the biliary canaliculus or the tight junctions around it, or even precipitation of micellar bile salts in the biliary system. Those drugs which produce both cholestasis and evidence of liver cell damage, "cholestatic hepatitis", may have the added factor of inflammatory exudation and oedema mechanically compressing bile ducts within the portal areas.

In patients with liver cell damage due to drugs, again two patterns of damage are found. Firstly, widespread spotty liver cell damage and inflammatory changes in the portal tracts similar to the changes of infective hepatitis are typical of so-called drug hepatitis. Sometimes this type of reaction is thought—because of its rarity—to represent the effects of some inherent sensitivity of the patient to the drug or one of its metabolites. A second type of liver cell damage is associated with hepatic necrosis often found in one particular part of the liver lobule. It is known, for example, that centrilobular regions of hepatic lobule are particularly prone to damage from anoxia, and this may render them susceptible to the action of drugs which in sensitive patients may produce centrilobular necrosis. On the other hand, damage is sometimes peripheral rather than central, and on other occasions generalised or massive necrosis may lack any zonal pattern at all.

Drugs producing this type of damage may do so because of a hypersensitivity of the patient, but on the other hand it is thought that reactive metabolites or even the parent drug itself may bind (covalent binding) to important intracellular organelles, producing liver cell dysfunction and damage.

Therapeutic Principles

It is obviously important to detect any drug which may have been responsible for hepatic damage in a patient and to withdraw it. Unfortunately this is not always as easy as is thought, because the numbers of possible drugs are large and it may be difficult to unravel the effects of various drugs from those of any underlying disease. Great care is therefore required in documentation of drugs which a patient is taking, and precise details may require the help of relatives, the family doctor, district nurse, pharmacist etc.

Patients with cholestatic liver disease need careful investigation to make certain that drugs are responsible for their symptoms and not, for example, an unsuspected pancreatic cancer. Careful visualisation of the biliary tree, e.g. by ERCP or transhepatic cholangiography, possibly supplemented by needle biopsy, will therefore be required. Once a definite diagnosis of drug-induced biliary obstruction has been made, no treatment is known to increase the rate of resolution of the disorder other than stopping the offending drug. Care must be taken to make sure that the effects of complications of cholestasis such as steatorrhoea and various fat-soluble vitamin deficiencies do not become manifest by means of appropriate therapy. There is no evidence to suggest that corticosteroids increase the rate of normalisation of biliary obstruction, and in patients with chronic biliary obstruction they can be harmful.

Similar therapeutic principles apply to patients who have evidence of liver cell dysfunction caused by drugs. Distinction must be made between drug-induced disease and disease caused by agents such as the various hepatitis viruses or alcohol. The basis of treatment is the early detection and removal of causative drugs, and support for impaired liver cell function as previously described. Again, corticosteroids seem to have no place in this process.

It may well be possible to apply more specific therapy for some of the agents which cause a dose-related injury to liver cells, often with a zonal pattern of necrosis. This certainly is so for paracetamol poisoning.

Paracetamol Toxicity

This drug has gained great popularity as a mild analgesic but unfortunately poisoning has also become common, perhaps 10% of overdoses being due to this drug. It is also a component (together with dextropropoxyphene) of Distalgesic, which again has become disproportionately popular as an agent for self-poisoning.

Paracetamol damages the liver to produce a predominantly centrilobular hepatic necrosis. As little as 6 g paracetamol (12 tablets) may cause liver damage, and death may occur after 15 g. Toxicity is increased in patients taking enzyme-inducing agents such as alcohol because toxicity is caused by the production of a reactive metabolite (a quinone-imine) rather than the parent drug. This binds irreversibly to organelles within the hepatocytes. The toxic metabolite is normally inactivated by hepatic reduced glutathione, but with a large overdose this protective mechanism is overwhelmed. Cysteamine, methionine and N-acetylcysteine have been used to treat severe paracetamol poisoning and probably act by repleting hepatic glutathione.

Assessment

The early symptoms are nausea, vomiting and abdominal discomfort. There are no abnormal physical signs during the first 24 hours. Abdominal pain and tenderness, jaundice, a bleeding tendency and elevation of the aspartate and alanine transaminases are deferred for 2–3 days, and in severe cases fulminant hepatic failure with high mortality may supervene.

Assessment of severity cannot necessarily be related to the number of tablets taken, and measurement of blood levels is the only reliable measure of likely severity. Levels of paracetamol >200 μg/ml at 4 h after ingestion, and of 50 μg/ml at 12 h with appropriate levels at intervening times allow the recognition of a group of patients likely to sustain severe liver damage.

Non-drug Treatment

The stomach should be washed out using a wide-bore gastric tube, and blood is taken into a heparinised container for immediate determination of paracetamol levels. It is critical that as near an accurate estimate as possible is made of the time of the overdose. Only patients who are seen within 10 h of the taking of the drug are suitable for treatment.

Drug Treatment

1. Methionine—this is comparatively ineffective but has the advantage that it is less toxic than other drugs and is given orally as soon as the diagnosis is made, via an indwelling gastric tube. Dose: 2.5 g.

2. Cysteamine—this was the standard antidote in patients seen within 10 h of poisoning, providing blood levels were predictive of hepatic damage. It probably restores depleted hepatic glutathione and may act as a precursor or alternative substrate for toxic metabolites. Cysteamine is given i.v. 2 g followed by 1.2 g infused over 20 h. It is often accompanied by unpleasant side-effects such as nausea and vomiting. However, no long-term toxic effects have been noted.

3. N-acetylcysteine (NAC)—marketed originally as 'Airbron', a mucolytic agent. NAC is now available for i.v. use in the treatment of acute paracetamol

poisoning. The same restrictions on its use in relation to time following poisoning and blood levels exist as for cysteamine. NAC is a sulphydryl (SH) donor, and there is also some evidence that it inhibits microsomal oxidation of paracetamol. An initial dose of 150 mg/kg is given i.v. over 15 min, followed by 50 mg/kg body weight in 500 ml dextrose over 4 h and 100 mg/kg body weight in 1 litre of 5% dextrose over the next 16 h, giving a total dose of 300 mg/kg body weight in 20 h. Hypokalaemia is a possible side-effect of treatment, and the plasma level should be carefully monitored.

In a study of 67 patients with paracetamol poisoning and the predicted probability of developing liver disease, an excellent result was obtained if treatment with NAC was given within 10 h.

Further Reading

Viral hepatitis

Sherlock S (ed) (1980) Virus hepatitis. Clin Gastroenterol 9(1) Saunders, London Philadelphia Toronto

Primary biliary cirrhosis

Long RG, Scheuer PJ, Sherlock S (1977) Presentation and course of asymptomatic primary biliary cirrhosis. Gastroenterology 72: 1204–1207
Sherlock S, Scheuer PJ (1973) The presentation and diagnosis of 100 patients with primary biliary cirrhosis. N Engl J Med 289: 674–678

Haemochromatosis

Powell LW, Bassett ML, Halliday JW (1980) Haemochromatosis: 1980 update. Gastroenterology 78: 374–381

Alcoholic liver disease

Lieber CS (1978) Pathogenesis and early diagnosis of alcoholic liver injury N Engl J Med 298: 888–893

Liver cell failure

Green JRB (1977) Mechanism of hypogonadism in cirrhotic males. Gut 18: 843–853
Zieve L (1979) Hepatic encephalopathy: summary of present knowledge with an elaboration on recent developments. In: Pepper H, Schaffner F (eds) Progress in liver disease, vol 6. Grune and Stratton, New York
Jenkins PJ, Wilkins R (1980) Fulminant viral hepatitis. Clin Gastroenterol 9(1) 171–189

Variceal haemorrhages

Terblanche J, Northover JMA, Bornman P et al. (1979) A prospective evaluation of injection sclerotherapy in the treatment of acute bleeding from oesophageal varices. Surgery 85: 239–245
Sherlock S (1978) Portal circulation and portal hypertension. Gut 19: 70–83

Ascites

Sherlock S, Senewiratne B, Scott A, Walker JG (1966) Complications of diuretic therapy in hepatic cirrhosis. Lancet I: 1049–1052

Wilkinson SP (1977) Liver disease and the kidney. Medicine (Lond, 2nd series) 29: 1647–1652

Drugs and liver disease

Read AE (1979) The liver and drugs. In: Wright R, Alberti KGMM, Karran S, Millward Sadler GH (eds) Liver and biliary disease. Saunders, London, p 822

Cholestasis

Boyer JL (1980, 2nd quarter) Cholestasis—concepts of pathogenesis based on current models of bile secretion. Hepatology Rapid Literature Review Short Form. Falk Foundation, p ix

9 Pancreatic Disease
R. A. Mountford

Acute Pancreatitis

Pathophysiology

Over 50% of acute pancreatitis is due to biliary tract disease. In the majority of the remainder no aetiological factor is discovered but a significant proportion are related to alcoholism. Other causes include mumps, hyperparathyroidism, carcinoma and drugs.

Treatment

Supportive Measures—Non-drug

During the first 6 h of illness 20%–30% of circulating blood volume may be lost, and this loss may continue. Therefore rapid fluid replacement is necessary, ideally with monitoring of central venous pressure or even a Swan-Ganz catheter.

Electrolytes should be monitored, including the serum calcium—severe hypocalcaemia carries a grave prognosis.

Parenteral nutrition is worth considering in patients who are initially malnourished, especially deteriorated alcoholics and those in whom ileus is prolonged. Temporary glucose intolerance may require addition of insulin when high concentrations of dextrose are infused.

Nasogastric suction is traditional, although there is little evidence that it benefits the patient.

Supportive Measures—Drugs

Adequate pain relief is critical and intravenous diamorphine may be required. Pethidine may elevate serum amylase, so blood samples should be dispatched before narcotic drugs are given.

Routine prophylactic use of antibiotics is not recommended. However, should infection, e.g. pneumonia, supervene, suitable antibiotic therapy is indicated. Heart failure may clearly require digitalisation, and some authorities use this drug routinely in patients over 60 years of age. Similarly, hypotension with oliguria despite adequate fluid replacement can be treated with infusions of dobutamine or dopamine; frusemide should be given if oliguria persists.

Many patients are found to be hypoxic, and unless there is coexisting respiratory disease, oxygen should be administered by mask. It is wise to monitor the arterial blood gases.

Specific Measures—Non-drug

Rises in serum amylase occur in a number of acute intra-abdominal events, including perforated peptic ulcer and small bowel infarction. Patients presenting with this biochemical finding and pronounced clinical signs of peritonism may reasonably be submitted to laparotomy. If the patient in fact is suffering grave acute pancreatitis, laparotomy is not in itself associated with increased mortality.

Fluid collections in the peritoneal cavity should be removed and lavage carried out. This manoeuvre is apparently beneficial. This has led to the suggestion that peritoneal lavage be performed in patients with acute pancreatitis not submitted to laparotomy; that is to say, by means of a peritoneal dialysis catheter. This appears a reasonable approach, although controlled data are lacking.

If acute pancreatitis is discovered at laparotomy, most surgeons would resect clearly necrotic portions of the gland. Total pancreatectomy in the acute situation has been performed but has not enjoyed general acceptance. Some surgeons will perform cholecystectomy and exploration of the common duct if gall-stones are found at operation and are suspected to be causative. Acute pancreatitis has until recently been regarded as a contra-indication to ERCP; however, apparent benefit has been claimed if ERCP is performed early in the disease. If gall-stones are found in the common duct, a papillotomy can be performed and stones removed from the common duct. This procedure has not gained full acceptance either.

Specific Measures—Drugs

There is no clear clinical benefit associated with the routine use of aprotinin (Trasylol), anticholinergics, glucagon or steroids. This is despite animal work suggesting efficacy if some of these agents are given either before or shortly after the onset of experimental pancreatitis.

Prevention of Further Attacks

This depends upon removal of the causative agent. Thus it is rational to urge the alcoholic patient to desist from his habit, to treat hyperlipidaemia and hyperparathyroidism, to withdraw any drugs which might be implicated and to remove gall-stones.

Complications

Following an attack of acute pancreatitis, a mass frequently develops and may become palpable on abdominal examination. A solid mass of inflammatory tissue, a phlegmon, may be demonstrated by ultrasound or CT scanning. This will often settle without specific therapy. However, careful monitoring should be performed in any patient with persistent abdominal pain, tenderness and a palpable mass (especially if there is evidence of progressive enlargement) or with prolonged elevation of serum amylase. This is probably most easily done by serial ultrasound scans. A collection of fluid, or pseudocyst, may form, most frequently in the lesser sac. Small cysts usually resorb spontaneously, but rarely they may discharge into a hollow viscus, most frequently the stomach, with spontaneous resolution. However, large and particularly expanding lesions are associated with a risk of erosion of surrounding structures, occasionally with life-threatening haemorrhage.

Percutaneous drainage of such pseudocysts has been described, and this procedure warrants consideration. If sufficient time has elapsed for the wall of the cavity to have matured into firm fibrous and granulation tissue, surgical drainage should be considered. This is usually in the form of marsupialisation of the sac wall into the posterior wall of the stomach.

The most dreaded complication of acute pancreatitis is abscess formation. This should be considered if the patient remains ill and develops a high swinging fever with leucocytosis. If infection is with gas-forming organisms, the diagnosis can occasionally be made on plain abdominal radiographs. Multiple gas-filled spaces will be seen, and if barium is placed in the stomach, it will frequently be demonstrated displaced anteriorly. The abscess cavity consists of pus, blood, debris and necrotic pancreatic tissue. The abscess may enlarge and erode surrounding structures, often with multiple tracks. The condition is uniformly fatal unless treated surgically. At operation the abscess is explored, all tracks opened, and adequate drainage instituted under antibiotic cover.

Chronic Pancreatitis

Chronic pancreatitis is associated with varying degrees of exocrine and endocrine failure.

"Pancreatic diabetes" is managed in the conventional manner. Usually the degree of glucose intolerance is mild and readily controlled. Occasionally the diabetes is "brittle" with violent swings of blood glucose. This has been attributed to coexisting abnormalities of glucagon secretion.

The management of steatorrhoea related to pancreatic exocrine failure has been dealt with elsewhere in this book (Chapter 3).

If chronic pancreatitis is painless, treatment of diabetes and enzyme supplements, with or without H_2 blockers or antacids, are all that is required. Many patients, however, have severe and often intractable pain, which can prove very difficult to manage. This type of disease occurs particularly in alcoholics. If such patients abstain for a few months, they may become pain free. Those who do not lose their pain, despite abstinence, and those who continue to drink and to suffer pain, form a very difficult group to manage. Suicide and narcotic addiction are not uncommon in this group. Unfortunately there is evidence that structural damage to the gland may be progressive despite abstinence, once the process is established. Coeliac ganglionectomy only renders a minority of patients pain free, and the effect of this procedure is frequently only temporary. Surgical relief of pain may be sought. It is necessary to delineate the pancreatic duct, either pre-operatively by means of ERCP, or intra-operatively. The purpose of this is to establish whether the disease is total or localised and whether the duct is narrowed or obstructed in one or more sites.

Localised disease may be treated by partial pancreatectomy—resection of the tail or body and tail—or by a Whipple's procedure. Unfortunately, disease may be more widespread than is indicated radiologically, and it frequently progresses in the unresected moiety of the gland. Drainage procedures may give temporary relief, but often further strictures develop, even if the patient has stopped drinking.

These lesser procedures are assayed in order to avoid total pancreatectomy, which is a formidable undertaking with a high operative mortality. Furthermore it is inevitably followed by diabetes, which carries a very high mortality in unreformed alcoholics. Hence much effort has been expended in attempting to preserve islet cell function, including transplant techniques. None of these is generally available.

Carcinoma of the Pancreas

Peri-ampullary carcinoma is treated by means of the Whipple procedure if metastases have not already occurred. If metastases have been demonstrated, attempts may be made to palliate the disease. Specifically, attempts may be made to relieve jaundice. This can be done by endoscopic sphincterotomy, with or without emplacement of a tube prosthesis to maintain drainage. Alternatively, a tube may be placed through the growth using the percutaneous transhepatic route. These procedures are still under assessment. Surgical palliation is by biliary diversion. If there is a risk of duodenal obstruction, a gastroenterostomy is also performed.

Carcinoma of the head, body and tail of the gland carries a very poor prognosis, median survival being about 5 months from diagnosis. Many surgeons have abandoned attempts to resect such growths, contenting themselves with "triple by-pass" (as above) procedures for palliation. On the other hand, some surgeons have claimed better survival with more extensive resections. This awaits further confirmation.

Endocrine-Secreting Tumours of the Pancreas

Insulinoma

About 75% of patients with endogenous hyperinsulinism have a solitary β-cell adenoma. This is curable by resection. Vigorous attempts should be made to localise the tumour pre-operatively. They tend to be vascular tumours and may be readily demonstrated on angiography. Alternatively, a regional venous sampling method can be used, determining insulin concentrations at various points in the splenic, superior mesenteric and portal vessels. Access to the portal system is achieved pre-operatively by the percutaneous transhepatic route.

The remaining cases are due to diffuse islet cell hypoplasia or carcinoma. The former is a condition largely of children and total or subtotal pancreatectomy may be required for clinical relief of symptoms.

Insulin-secreting islet cell carcinoma is an aggressive growth which has frequently metastasised by the time of diagnosis. If secondaries are confirmed, laparotomy is not justified. The metastases frequently secrete large quantities of insulin. Treatment is directed towards mitigating the resulting hypoglycaemia. Diazoxide is effective in an initial dose of 5 mg/kg daily, divided into two or three doses. This is increased up to a maximal adult dose of 1 g daily. Hypertrichosis may be a troublesome side-effect. Fluid retention frequently occurs, necessitating the concomitant administration of a diuretic. Steroids may enhance the effect of the drug. If diazoxide is ineffective or becomes so (tachyphylaxis may be a problem), an alternative is streptozotocin. This is given in a dose of 1–2 g/m^2 weekly for 4 weeks by intravenous injection. The main side-effect is nephrotoxicity, although liver damage has also been reported.

Zollinger-Ellison Syndrome

Gastrinomas present with intractable, recurrent peptic ulceration of the upper gastrointestinal tract or with steatorrhoea, or both. Approximately 25% of patients have multiple endocrine adenomatosis.

A solitary pancreatic gastrinoma occurs in less than 30% of cases, and of these more than one-third are malignant. Surgical resection may be curative. Seventy percent of patients are found to have multifocal disease, and of these, two-thirds have metastases at presentation. Until recently this group of patients were treated by total gastrectomy. Many authorities now prefer to use H^2 blockers, although large doses may be required (up to 8 g/day of cimetidine).

Vipoma (Werner-Morrison Syndrome)

In 1959 Werner and Morrison described a syndrome of watery diarrhoea, hypokalaemia and achlorhydria. Up to 5 litres of watery stool may be passed every 24 h, giving a clinical picture similar to cholera.

Of a review of 54 cases, 43 were associated with pancreatic tumours, 23 of which were benign. Extra-pancreatic tumours occur in about 10%. Within the pancreas, most occur in body or tail and are single, usually greater than 3 cm in diameter. They are well circumscribed and can be enucleated from the surrounding pancreatic tissue.

Glucagonoma

This rare syndrome is characterised by diabetes, anaemia and a migratory erythematous skin rash with skin necrosis and crusting. The tumour is highly malignant, although local resection has been reported. Chemotherapy with streptozotocin or L-asparaginase may be effective. Somatostatin may have a role in irresectable cases.

Further Reading

Cuschieri A, Wormsley KG (1980) The pancreas. In: Bouchier IAD (ed) Recent advances in gastroenterology, vol 4. Churchill Livingstone, Edinburgh London New York, pp 223–249
Keynes WM, Keith RG (1981) The pancreas. Tutorials in postgraduate medicine. Heinemann Medical, London

10 Tropical Diseases Affecting the Gastrointestinal Tract and Liver

M. M. A. Homeida and T. K. Daneshmend

Amoebic Dysentery

Pathophysiology

Amoebiasis is caused by the protozoon *Entamoeba histolytica*. Although multiple organs may be involved, the colon is the main and initial site of infection. Amoebiasis has a world-wide distribution, being extremely common in the tropics and subtropics—particularly where sanitary conditions are poor. Morbidity and mortality from amoebiasis show considerable geographical variation.

The disease is contracted by ingestion of *Entamoeba* cysts in contaminated food or drink. In the human intestine these cysts release four-nucleated trophozoites which divide to form uninucleate trophozoites which are the motile and pathogenic (vegetative) form of the organism. The trophozoites invade the colonic mucosa and produce colonies in the gut wall which ulcerate. Some trophozoites become encysted, are shed in the stools and perpetuate the life cycle by further faecal–oral spread. The viability of these trophozoites in the colon depends on the presence of bacteria with which they live in symbiosis, e.g. *Escherichia coli* and *Enterobacteria aerogenes*.

The incubation period is variable and often difficult to ascertain. Infection with *Entamoeba histolytica* may produce an extremely variable clinical picture, ranging from severe diarrhoea with systemic upset similar to frank ulcerative colitis, to an asymptomatic cyst-carrier state. In acute amoebic dysentery half the cases have a sudden onset and the incubation period may be only 10 days. Often the development of dysenteric symptoms is insidious, with abdominal colic, headache, nausea, anorexia and malaise. Patients are said to be characteristically afebrile, though this is by no means invariable. The stools contain mucus and streaks of blood. In the chronic cyst-carrier state a minority experience the symptoms of alternating diarrhoea and constipation. However, the clinical picture does not correlate with the presence of amoebic cysts in the stool.

Amoebic colitis is the result of invasive ulcers produced by the trophozoites throughout the colon but especially the caecum and descending colon. The ulcers may become confluent by lateral spread in the submucosa. These ulcers have undermined edges, and in contrast to ulcerative colitis the colonic mucosa between these ulcers appears normal.

The diagnosis is made by finding *Entamoeba histolytica* trophozoites in a fresh stool specimen, colonic scrapings or a rectal biopsy specimen. The carrier state is diagnosed by finding *Entamoeba* cysts in the stools.

Therapeutic Principles

The aim of treatment is to eradicate both the vegetative and cyst forms of the amoeba.

Drug Treatment

Metronidazole is now the drug of choice in the treatment of acute amoebic dysentery. However, recent reports, notably from India, have recorded treatment failures with this drug and suggested supplementation with other agents. The standard dose is metronidazole 800 mg three times per day for 10 days. In children a dose of 50 mg metronidazole per kilogram per day is given for 10 days. This course will cure up to 90% of all patients. However, at this dose of metronidazole, nausea, vomiting, giddiness and lassitude often develop and treatment may have to be stopped. Therefore a shorter 5-day course of metronidazole followed by diloxanide furoate 500 mg daily for 10 days may be better tolerated and equally effective.

Tinidazole, a 5-nitroimidazole similar to metronidazole, given in a single daily dose of 2 g for 3 days, appears to be as effective as metronidazole with the advantage of being better tolerated. Alternatively, tetracycline or oxytetracycline 250 mg four times per day for 10 days may be given following a 5-day course of metronidazole. These antibiotics have no direct amoebicidal action but act by killing the bacteria with which the amoebae live in symbiosis. In an especially severe attack of amoebic dysentery in a child or adult, tetracycline 250 mg four times per day should be given concurrently with metronidazole for 10 days. A course of diloxanide furoate may be added to this regime if required.

Emetine and dehydroemetine hydrochloride have largely been replaced by the less toxic agents mentioned above and are now rarely used. These drugs have a low therapeutic ratio. Toxicity includes nausea, vomiting, hypotension, chest pain, tachycardia and dyspnoea.

Iodoquinol and clioquinol are derivatives of 8-hydroxyquinoline and have been widely used in mild acute amoebiasis and in "traveller's diarrhoea". However, in view of the definite link between clioquinol and subacute myelo-optic neuropathy, their use for such trivial infections cannot be recommended.

Treatment of the Carrier State

Diloxanide furoate 500 mg three times daily for 10 days is the drug of choice. Metronidazole and tinidazole are of little use in treating the cyst-carrier state. At least six stool samples after the course of treatment should be without cysts to establish a cure.

Amoebic Liver Abscess

Pathophysiology

In amoebic infection the liver is the most commonly involved extra-intestinal organ. Vegetative amoebae migrate from the intestine via the portal vein and cause amoebic abscess, which is in the right lobe of the liver in 90% of patients. Usually the amoebic liver abscess is solitary, but a quarter of patients have multiple abscesses. At presentation amoebic dysentery is present in less than half the patients and some may be unaware of any previous episode of amoebic colitis. The patient is usually ill with a low-grade or high fever, anorexia, weight loss and, uncommonly, jaundice. Pain in the right side of the abdomen and tender hepatomegaly occur when the abscess reaches the liver surface. Elevation of the right hemidiaphragm, pleural effusion and atelectasis occur often. Amoebic liver abscess may have an unusual presentation and be initially misdiagnosed because of a hepatocellular or cholestatic pattern of jaundice, possibly with hepatic encephalopathy. Laboratory features are leucocytosis, moderate anaemia and raised alkaline phosphatase. Serology is extremely helpful in invasive (extra-intestinal) amoebic disease and the complement fixation test is positive in almost all cases of amoebic liver abscess.

Therapeutic Principles

Abscesses are demonstrated in the liver by an ultrasound or radio-isotope scan. The diagnosis is confirmed by the aspiration of brownish 'pus' in which vegetative amoebae are seen.

Drug Treatment

Metronidazole given as an oral dose of 800 mg three times a day for 10 days is the treatment of choice. As with amoebic dysentery, there is a high failure rate in those who have acquired the disease in India. Tinidazole 2 g daily for 3 days is as effective as metronidazole in adults and has also been used in children at a dose of 50 mg/kg per day for 3–5 days. In the vast majority of patients successful resolution of the abscess can be effected with drugs only, though it may take months for a space-occupying defect on liver scan to resolve. Unfortunately most serological tests remain positive after successful treatment and therefore cannot be used to monitor the resolution of amoebic liver abscess.

Non-drug Treatment

Needle aspiration may be necessary for a large abscess in a very ill patient. Indications for needle aspiration are (a) tender hepatomegaly with failure of the above drugs, (b) local tenderness, oedema and fluctuation suggesting that the abscess may be pointing to the surface and (c) elevation of the right hemidiaphragm. Each aspiration should be limited to a litre and may be repeated at intervals. Haemorrhage and secondary infection are complications of aspiration.

Open drainage of amoebic abscess may be necessary if (a) the pus is too viscous for aspiration, (b) the volume daily aspirated is in excess of 0.5–1 litre, (c) secondary infection is present, (d) there is rupture of the abscess and (e) there is a danger of rupture.

Amoebic Peritonitis

Pathophysiology

This results from (a) passage of organisms through a "blotting-paper" like colon or (b) colonic perforation, which may be peritoneal or retroperitoneal and may result in localisation of the disease or be accompanied by a faecal peritonitis.

Usually the perforation is insidious, with minimal pain and some tenderness over the colon. When the process is chronic the picture may resemble tuberculous peritonitis. Paracentesis may aid in diagnosis if amoebae are found.

Treatment

Supportive measures such as intravenous fluids and nasogastric suction are necessary. Metronidazole should be given parenterally along with a broad-spectrum antibiotic. Surgery is only of help when the perforation is sudden.

About half the patients with amoebic peritonitis succumb. In patients with insidious onset surgery is invariably fatal.

Amoeboma

Pathophysiology

Amoeboma is formed when a granulomatous reaction follows localised ulceration or penetration of tissues by amoebae. The caecum and recto-sigmoid colon are common sites and the length of bowel affected varies. Multiple amoebomas may be present. Clinically amoeboma presents as a painful tender mass and causes intestinal obstruction by projecting into the bowel or by stricture formation. It is often misdiagnosed as carcinoma of the colon or an appendix mass. Serology is usually positive, stools may be negative for amoebae or cysts, sigmoidoscopy may show ulcers and barium enema may show a stricture with smooth edges.

Treatment

Treatment is with metronidazole as for amoebic colitis and resolution is usually complete within a week.

Intestinal Schistosomiasis

Pathophysiology

Intestinal schistosomiasis is caused mainly by three species of schistosome (trematodes or liver flukes): *Schistosoma mansoni, S. japonicum* and *S. haematobium*. Of these the first two produce significant intestinal pathology, while *S. haematobium* causes mainly genito-urinary schistosomiasis. Schistosomiasis affects over 200 million individuals world-wide. Disease with *S. haematobium* and *S. mansoni* is widespread in Africa and the Middle East, while *S. mansoni* only is found in Central and South America and certain Caribbean islands. *S. japonicum* infection is endemic in the Far East, China, the Philippines and Indonesia. Schistosomiasis is found mainly in rural and agricultural communities. Poor sanitation, contaminated water and specific snail hosts are necessary for the persistence of schistosomiasis in the community.

The complex life cycle consists of a sexual generation in the human host and an asexual multiplicative generation in a snail host. Adult worms live in sexual pairs in the human portal venous system, the mesenteric plexus (*S.*

japonicum) and the haemorrhoidal plexus (*S. mansoni*). These worm pairs live for about 5 years and each pair may produce 300–3000 eggs per day. These are laid in the submucosal layer of the gut wall, where half of them find their way into the gut lumen. After being shed the eggs hatch on entering fresh water, and the larval stage (miracidium) invades the snail host. Within the snail many new cercariae are produced and liberated. These cercariae swim about and penetrate intact human skin, after which they are carried to the portal venous system via the bloodstream and the life cycle is completed. The eggs which are not shed lodge in human tissues and excite a vigorous inflammatory reaction and granuloma formation. Ova travelling to the liver in the branches of the portal vein give rise to the main complication of intestinal schistosomiasis, namely periportal hepatic fibrosis with resultant presinusoidal portal hypertension.

Infections with schistosomes may be completely asymptomatic. Four or six weeks after infection with *S. mansoni* or *S. intercalatum* there may be a generalised allergic reaction with malaise, fever, myalgia, urticaria and eosinophilia. This is followed, months or years later, by dysenteric symptoms: diarrhoea with mucus and blood, and epigastric pain. The presence of visible colonic lesions on sigmoidoscopy varies in different parts of the world. A quarter of patients with *S. mansoni* infection in Egypt develop polyposis of the colon. In the chronic stage the patient may be anaemic and emaciated. Extensive colonic polyposis is responsible for blood and protein loss, which contribute to the anaemia and hypoproteinaemia. With progressive development of hepatic involvement there is hepatosplenomegaly and evidence of portal hypertension. Many patients present at the stage of marked portal hypertension with haematemesis and melaena. At this late stage the liver may be shrunken and the spleen enlarged. In compensated cases of hepatosplenic schistosomiasis hepatocyte function is preserved in contrast to the hepatocellular failure present in cirrhosis of the liver.

Therapeutic Principles

The diagnosis is confirmed by finding the characteristic schistosome eggs in the stools or in a rectal scraping or biopsy. Though the main pathology results from a reaction to the eggs, treatment is directed towards killing the adult worm pairs and so stopping further laying of eggs. Patients with anaemia, emaciation and hypoproteinaemia require blood transfusion, and dietary supplements of vitamins and minerals. The presence of hepatic involvement limits the use of certain drugs.

Drug Treatment

Until recently the development of schistosomicides has been slow. One of the major problems is deciding which patients with schistosomiasis should be given the drugs since most live in endemic areas and become reinfected rapidly. Clearly, patients with no further risk of reinfection should be treated and a complete cure aimed for.

Until recently the most widely used drug was niridazole (Ambilhar). The oral dose is 25 mg/kg daily for 7 days or 20 mg/kg daily for 10 days. It is most active against *S. haematobium* infections and is least active against *S. japonicum*. Toxic reactions with niridazole affect the nervous system and result in acute psychoses, hallucinations and convulsions. These prevent the use of this drug in mass chemotherapy campaigns. The neurotoxic manifestations are especially likely in hepatocellular dysfunction or when portal systemic shunting exists, whereby niridazole may by-pass the liver, avoiding hepatic conjugation.

Oxamniquine (Vansil, Mansil) is the drug of choice for *S. mansoni* infection, though there is marked variation in response to the drug in different areas. In South America a total oral oxamniquine dose of 20 mg/kg appears to be effective. However, in Africa satisfactory results are only obtained at a total oral dose of 60 mg/kg. The dose is divided and given over 2 days. These differences in dose requirements of oxamniquine have not yet been explained. The drug appears to be less effective in children than adults. Side-effects tend to be few and non-serious.

Hycanthone is also effective in the treatment of *S. mansoni* and *S. haematobium*, but not *S. japonicum*. It has to be given by intramuscular injection in a dose of 2.5–3 mg/kg. However, there are serious side-effects, in particular hepatotoxicity. Severe anaemia, malnutrition and pregnancy are also contra- indications to the use of hycanthone.

Praziquantel, a new isoquinoline compound, is highly effective against all three species of schistosome. A single oral dose of 40 mg/kg is required for *S. haematobium* and *S. mansoni*. For *S. japonicum* the effective oral dose is 30 mg/ kg on two occasions 4 h apart or 20 mg/kg on three occasions 4 h apart. Side-effects are infrequent and transient.

Metriphonate is effective only against *S. haematobium* and is given in doses of 7.5 mg/kg once every 2–4 weeks on two to three occasions.

The bivalent antimony compounds (sodium antimony tartrate, stibocaptate and stibophen) are now seldom used and have largely been replaced by the newer relatively non-toxic drugs mentioned above. Occasionally they are used in the treatment of *S. japonicum* infection, though praziquantel is now the drug of choice. Sibocaptate is given in a total dose of 50 mg/kg (maximum dose of 2.5 g). The total dose is divided into five equal injections given weekly. Adverse effects following such treatment are many and severe: painful injection site, vomiting, abdominal pain, myalgia, bradycardia, hypotension and cardiac dysrhythmia.

Non-drug Treatment

Mechanical removal of the worms from the portal venous system has been used in individual cases. Antimony potassium tartrate is administered to induce migration of the worms into the portal veins. Adult worms are then trapped using a filter. This technique is of very limited value in the treatment of schistosomiasis.

Complications

Management of Oesophageal Variceal Haemorrhage

Variceal haemorrhage is a consequence of increasing portal hypertension in the hepatosplenic form of schistosomiasis. Adequate blood and fluid replacement are the mainstay of treatment and in the younger patient Pitressin may be of value in controlling haemorrhage. Patients with hepatosplenic schistosomiasis tolerate variceal bleeding better than patients with hepatic cirrhosis due to the relative preservation of hepatocellular function and younger age. Those patients who continue to have variceal haemorrhage on conservative management may be considered for endoscopic variceal sclerotherapy or surgical portosystemic shunts. Patients should be carefully selected for surgical portosystemic shunts, and the procedure appears to be better tolerated by such patients than by cirrhotics.

Intestinal Worms

Introduction

The clinically important worms causing intestinal disease belong mainly to the classes Nematoda and Cestoda. Nematodes of various genera result in intestinal infection in man: ankylostomiasis (hookworm disease), ascariasis (roundworm disease), trichuriasis (whipworm disease), strongyloidiasis (threadworm disease) and enterobiasis (pinworm disease). The commoner Cestoda infections in man are taeniasis (tapeworm disease) and hymenolepiasis (dwarf tapeworm disease). Fasciolopsiasis (intestinal and liver fluke infection) is caused by trematodes, a class which includes schistosomes. The latter cause intestinal disease but the worms do not live in the gut lumen. Schistosomiasis has been discussed earlier.

Infection with these worms has a world-wide distribution and in most tropical areas the vast majority of the population is infected. Infection with intestinal tapeworms remains endemic due to poor personal and environmental hygiene. Though the mortality from these diseases is low, the morbidity is long and affects physical and intellectual performance.

Ankylostomiasis (Hookworm Disease)

Ankylostoma duodenale or *Necator americanus* infections affect most of the populations living in tropical countries. Hookworm infections may be present in a quarter of the world's population according to one estimate. *Necator* appears to be less pathogenic than *Ankylostoma*, though both parasites are now equally widely distributed in the tropics.

The adult worms, about 1 cm long, rely on suction to anchor themselves to the duodenal and jejunal villi. The symptoms depend upon the amount of blood loss from anchor sites. This is determined by the worm load, which if heavy, results in anaemia and hypoproteinaemia. Each female hookworm produces between 10 000 and 30 000 eggs per day, which on moist soil hatch into larvae. These larvae remain viable in the soil for several months and penetrate human skin on contact. They migrate via the heart and lungs to the trachea and are swallowed and reach the jejunum and duodenum 5 days after skin penetration. *Ankylostoma* but not *Necator* can also infect by the oral route.

Abdominal symptoms of discomfort, occasional diarrhoea and flatulence occur a few weeks after a sizeable infection. As the hookworm load increases, a hypochromic, microcytic anaemia appears after 3–6 months, followed by signs of hypoproteinaemia.

Diagnosis is made by identifying the eggs in faeces. The aims of treatment are to correct the iron deficiency and to kill and expel the worms. Iron deficiency almost always responds fully to oral iron, and iron infusion is rarely necessary. Blood transfusion is seldom needed even for severe cases and carries a high risk of producing cardiac failure.

Treatment

Bephenium hydroxynaphthoate is the drug of choice for both *Ankylostoma* and *Necator* infections, though it is more effective against the former. The dose is 5 g orally after an overnight fast on three successive days. A syrup formulation is available for children. Side-effects are occasional nausea and vomiting.

Mebendazole is a broad-spectrum antihelminthic with few side-effects. The dose is 100 mg twice daily for 3 days, though a failure rate of 15% has been recorded with this regime. Mebendazole is also effective against *Ascaris lumbricoides* and therefore appropriate when ankylostomiasis and ascariasis both infect the same patient.

Pyrantel embonate given as a single dose of 750 mg or 1 g appears to be as effective as bephenium hydroxynaphthoate.

Tetrachlorethylene given in a dose of 0.12 ml/kg body weight (maximum 5 ml per dose) after an overnight fast is an effective and cheap alternative to the above. Two or three doses may be required at 4-day intervals. It should not be given to patients with liver disease. The side-effects are nausea, vomiting and epigastric discomfort.

Ascariasis (Roundworm Infection)

Man is infected with *Ascaris lumbricoides* by ingesting the eggs in contaminated vegetables and water. The ova release larvae in the small intestine which burrow through the gut wall and reach the lungs via the portal blood and right atrium.

They migrate from the alveoli to the larynx and pharynx. They are then swallowed and again enter the small intestine where they mature and start producing ova.

On rare occasions larvae enter the systemic circulation and can cause symptoms in any part of the body. Passage through the lungs causes pneumonitis, cough and dyspnoea; the sputum may contain larvae. Mild infection is asymptomatic in the vast majority of cases. Heavy infection results in abdominal discomfort and colic. A bolus of worms rarely causes intestinal obstruction, and intussusception is sometimes seen in children. Though ascariasis does not cause malabsorption, malnutrition is often seen.

Diagnosis is made by finding ova in stool and sometimes adult worms are passed per rectum. A plain abdominal X-ray may show the worms; occasionally a barium meal may be helpful. There are no diagnostic serological tests. The aim of treatment is to eradicate the worms.

Treatment

Piperazine is the drug of choice. Adults should be given a single oral dose of 4 g. Children require 75 mg/kg body weight. A further dose may be necessary 1 week later. The side-effects are headache, dizziness and visual disturbance; convulsions are rare. Hepatic or renal disease and epilepsy are contra-indications.

Mebendazole is free of toxic effects and cure rates of 100% have been recorded. The dose is 100 mg twice daily on three successive days. In addition mebendazole may also eliminate coexistent hookworm infection.

Levamisole and tetramisole are effective against ascariasis and also ankylostomiasis and strongyloidiasis. For ascariasis, levamisole 2.5 mg/kg body weight is taken as a single oral dose. The side-effects of nausea, vomiting, abdominal discomfort and headaches are rare.

Trichuriasis (Whipworm Disease)

This is caused by *Trichuris trichiura*. These worms measure 3–5 cm and infect children more than adults. The simple life cycle is as follows: eggs are passed in stool, mature on soil and when swallowed hatch in the small intestine and caecum. The adult worms adhere to the mucosa of the ileum or caecum. Heavy infections cause chronic diarrhoea with mucus and blood in the stools. Abdominal pain is frequent and weight loss and anaemia may also occur.

Diagnosis is made by finding eggs in the stools and also at sigmoidoscopy by seeing the worms attached to the mucosa.

Treatment

Mebendazole is the agent of choice. For trichuriasis the recommended dose is 100 mg three times per day for 3 days. In some parts of the world a further course may be required. Addition of loperamide may improve cure rates.

Strongyloidiasis (Threadworm Disease)

The larvae of *Strongyloides stercoralis* are passed in stools and develop after 3 months into infective larvae which penetrate intact human skin. They travel via the bloodstream to the lungs, then through the trachea to the oesophagus and the small intestine, where they mature.

During the migratory phase of the larvae the symptoms are a serpiginous creeping skin eruption. Colicky abdominal pain with alternating diarrhoea and constipation occurs after some weeks. Heavy infection results in malabsorption and weight loss. Rarely death may result in patients with depressed immunity or when corticosteroids are given for presumed inflammatory bowel disease.

Diagnosis is established by finding larvae in fresh stool, and sometimes ova. Larvae and ova may be present in jejunal biopsy specimens or jejunal fluid. Serology for *S. stercoralis* is not diagnostic.

Treatment

Thiabendazole is the drug of choice. The dose is 25 mg/kg body weight twice a day on three consecutive days. The main side-effects are gastrointestinal (nausea, vomiting and diarrhoea); drowsiness and cardiovascular symptoms are occasionally seen. Mebendazole may be equally effective in a dose of 100 mg twice a day for 4 days.

Enterobiasis (Pinworm Disease)

This is caused by *Enterobius vermicularis* (also called *Oxyuris vermicularis* or threadworm). The infection is very common, particularly in children, usually affects whole families and may well be commoner outside the tropics. Ova are ingested in faecally contaminated food or water. The larvae hatch in the jejunum and pass to the colon via the ileum. The female worms shed ova which reach the peri-anal skin. Retroinfection and autoinfection are common.

Pruritus ani is the commonest symptom and often occurs at night. Scratching results is autoinfection and peri-anal dermatitis. Rarely vaginal discharge or prostatitis occurs. Gastrointestinal symptoms are usually mild. Diagnosis is confirmed by finding the ova or larvae near the anus. Ova may also be found beneath fingernails or in stools.

Treatment

Mebendazole is the drug of choice and a single oral dose of 100 mg repeated after 2 weeks is effective. Other drugs are: piperazine citrate 2 g per day for a week and pyrantel embonate 10 mg/kg body weight.

Usually the whole family needs to be treated, and advice about personal hygiene and toilet habits is as important as the drug treatment.

Taeniasis, Hymenolepiasis and Diphyllobothriasis

These tapeworm infections may be considered together as their parasitology and treatment are similar. *Taenia saginata* (beef tapeworm) and *T. solium* (pork tapeworm) infections are the commonest. Man is the definitive host and also acts as a casual intermediate host of *T. solium*. The common dwarf worms are *Hymenolepis nana* (dwarf tapeworm) and *H. diminuta* (rat tapeworm), which mainly infect children. *Diphyllobothrium latum* (fish tapeworm) is found in temperate and tropical regions, and can reach up to 10 m in length. The basic structure of these worms is of a small head and narrow neck (the scolex) followed by flat segments (the proglottids). Each segment contains male and female reproductive organs and produces eggs.

Ova of *T. solium* and *T. saginata*, when ingested by their animal hosts (pigs and cattle respectively), hatch into embryos in the gut and spread to other organs in the body. When raw beef infected with *T. saginata* is eaten by man it results in an adult worm in the intestine. When raw pork infected with *T. solium* is eaten, the infection is not limited to the intestine and the larvae spread to muscle, brain and subcutaneous tissue and encyst as cystircerci. The latter cause various neurological manifestations, e.g. epilepsy and intracranial hypertension. Fish tapeworm is acquired by eating infected salmon, pike or crustaceans which have been undercooked. *D. lateum* lives in the ileum.

Apart from some abdominal discomfort there are usually no symptoms from intestinal infection with tapeworms. Worm segments may be seen by the patient in stool, clothing or bedding. A megaloblastic anaemia may occur with *D. latum* due to ingestion of dietary vitamin B_{12} by the worm. *H. nana* causes abdominal pain, diarrhoea and weight loss when infection is severe.

Complications are rare except with *T. solium*, which causes cysticercosis. Rarely intestinal obstruction or perforation may be caused by the worms.

Diagnosis is made by finding and examining the segments and sometimes ova in stool. Haemagglutination tests may be of use in cysticercosis. Radiology may show calcified cysticerci in muscles. Brain cysticerci calcify very slowly.

Treatment

Niclosamide is the drug of choice for all tapeworm infections. A single oral dose of 2 g on an empty stomach is followed 2 h later by a saline purge of magnesium sulphate (30 ml). Niclosamide causes gastrointestinal upset and in *T. solium* infections carries the danger of causing cysticercosis if vomiting occurs. Consequently some authorities recommend mepacrine: 90 mg given as a single dose with an anti-emetic. Male fern extract has been superseded by niclosamide. Praziquantel and mebendazole have also been used with success. Cure is proven by identifying the scolex in stools. There is no effective treatment for cysticercosis.

Further Reading

Cook GC (1980) *Tropical gastroenterology*. Oxford University Press, Oxford
Harries J (1982) Amoebiasis: a review. J R Soc Med 75: 190–197
Marsden PD (ed) (1978) Intestinal parasites. Clin Gastroenterol 7(1) Saunders, London Philadelphia Toronto
Webbe G (1981) Schistosomiasis: some advances. Br Med J 283: 1104–1106

SECTION II

11 Clinical Pharmacological Considerations
C. J. C. Roberts

Introduction

Within the practice of the gastroenterologist there will be patients suffering from diseases of the alimentary tract and of the pancreas and hepatobiliary systems. The alimentary tract provides the portal of entry of most drugs and the liver is a major organ of their elimination; physiological alterations in gastrointestinal function and disease processes may therefore be expected to have a profound influence on the pharmacokinetics and actions of drugs. Therapy for conditions outside the gastrointestinal tract can be affected by gastrointestinal disturbance. Gastrointestinal disease not only influences drug action through altered absorption or elimination: alterations in body composition as a result of nutritional deficit or hepatic disease may also cause variations in the distribution characteristics of certain drugs which in turn may require changes in dose or dose interval. Both the liver and the alimentary tract provide important sites of drug interaction, and disease in these organs may affect the extent and significance of any such interaction. The liver is particularly sensitive to adverse drug effects, so that iatrogenic disease forms a significant proportion of any gastroenterologist's practice. Thus although the gastroenterologist uses specific drug therapy less frequently than do other specialists, he must always be aware firstly that the patient's disorder may be the result of previous medication and secondly that drug therapy of cardiovascular, respiratory, CNS or other types of disease may need to be adjusted in the presence of concurrent or intercurrent gastrointestinal disease. The aim of this chapter is to explore the special relationship of the alimentary tract and liver to clinical pharmacokinetics and drug action, and to provide examples of situations in which altered gastrointestinal function requires care in therapy for conditions outside the gastrointestinal tract.

Drug Absorption from the Gastrointestinal Tract

Theoretically absorption of drugs after oral administration can take place by four mechanisms: passive diffusion, active transport, filtration through pores and pinocytosis. Of these only the first two are of any practical significance.

Passive Diffusion

Most drugs enter the body by passive diffusion. The rate of diffusion is dependent on the concentration gradient across the epithelial membrane, and for absorption to proceed the drug must be in solution in the gastrointestinal lumen (aqueous phase) and must change to its lipid soluble phase in order to traverse the lipid cell membrane. Transport away from the epithelium in the blood requires reversion to the aqueous phase. The rate and extent of absorption of drug by passive diffusion will thus depend on gastrointestinal factors and drug factors.

Gastrointestinal Factors

Among the gastrointestinal factors affecting absorption of drugs by passive diffusion are the *surface area* of epithelium available—so that the major site of absorption is the small intestine, where the epithelial villi provide a huge surface area—and the time the drug spends in contact with the absorbing surface. This is important and depends on *gastrointestinal motility*. Because the small intestine is the major site of absorption of most drugs, slowed gastric emptying will tend to delay drug absorption and where transit through the small intestine is rapid the completeness of absorption of certain drugs may be reduced.

The presence of food in the gut lumen might be expected to reduce the rate of absorption of drugs by delaying gastric emptying, but it may enhance the systemic bioavailability of certain drugs, particularly those which undergo presystemic metabolism (see below). Indeed, the effect of food on the absorption of individual drugs may be quite unpredictable and specific studies of each drug are required if recommendation about dosing in relation to meals is to be made. Concurrent medications may prevent absorption of other drugs by chemically binding them within the gut lumen.

The water solubility and lipid:water partition coefficient of certain drugs are sensitive to changes in pH in the physiological range. Thus *changes in gut pH* might be expected to alter the absorption of these drugs. However, experimentation has not always supported the predicted outcome and pH changes are no longer considered as an important source of variability in drug absorption.

Some drugs undergo *metabolism in the gut wall*, where there are enzymes for acetylation, glucuronidation and sulphation. Variability in the activity of these enzyme systems will determine systemic bioavailability of certain drugs.

Drug Factors

The way in which a drug is *formulated* may have a profound effect on its absorption characteristics. The rate of release of active ingredient from a tablet or capsule will depend on its speed of disintegration, which in turn depends on the particle size and degree of compression used at manufacture. Where dissolution is slow and where drugs have been formulated in slow-release preparations the extent of absorption is highly dependent on gastrointestinal motility. The administration of drugs in slow-release form may be particularly unwise in the presence of acute gastrointestinal hurry.

All drugs that can be usefully absorbed must be *water soluble*; however, this is a factor that varies between drugs. Drugs with poor water solubility are more susceptible to variation in gastrointestinal function. *Lipid solubility* determines the ease with which the drug passes across the lipid cell membrane.

Water: lipid partition coefficient—Acidic drugs become ionised and more water soluble in an alkaline medium and vice versa. If the pKa of the drug is close to physiological pH then changes in that pH may materially alter the partition coefficient and therefore the absorption characteristics of the drug.

Active Transport

Very few drugs are absorbed actively. Naturally occurring substances such as amino acids, sugars and vitamins are, and it follows that drugs which resemble natural substances, such as methyldopa and L-dopa, may be absorbed by this mechanism.

The extent and rapidity of absorption of drugs from the gastrointestinal tract is thus determined by the interaction of these many factors. Highly soluble drugs will be less likely to suffer variability in absorption than poorly soluble compounds.

Drug Bioavailability

This term is used to describe the fraction of administered drug which enters the systemic circulation. It therefore incorporates loss of drug due to poor formulation and failure of drug absorption and loss of drug due to metabolism in the gut and liver.

Presystemic Metabolism ("First Pass Effect")

In order to gain access to the systemic circulation a drug, once absorbed, must pass via the portal venous system through the liver. Within the liver highly active extraction mechanisms and metabolic processes may remove and detoxify a proportion of the drug. The hepatic extraction ratio gives a guide to the extent of presystemic metabolism to which a drug is likely to be subject. This is the ratio of drug concentration in the hepatic vein to that entering the liver. For a drug which is fully absorbed from the gastrointestinal tract, systemic bioavailability is 100% minus the hepatic extraction ratio. Thus for a drug such as chlormethiazole the extraction ratio is on average 90% and the bioavailability 10%. There is usually wide interindividual variation in the activity of hepatic enzyme systems so that the range in bioavailability may be two- or threefold. Furthermore, the extent of first pass metabolism will be altered both by haemodynamic changes such as portosystemic shunting and possibly changes in portal blood flow and by the many factors which influence hepatic microsomal function such as enzyme inducing and inhibiting agents, acute and chronic liver disease and the ageing process.

Clinically Important Examples of Altered Drug Absorption and Bioavailability

Reduced Mucosal Surface

Diseases affecting small intestinal mucosa would be expected to reduce drug absorption (Table 11.1). However, the effect of coeliac disease and others is neither consistent nor predictable. Digoxin concentrations are reduced in coeliac disease, as are those of thyroxine, penicillin V and pivampicillin, and the absorption of amoxycillin, lincomycin and practolol is delayed. Indomethacin, aspirin and pivmecillinam levels are unaffected, whilst the bioavailability of co-trimoxazole, sodium fusidate and propranolol appears to be enhanced. The effect of Crohn's disease on drug absorption seems equally inconsistent, with levels of metronidazole and lincomycin being reduced, levels of clindamycin, co-trimoxazole and sodium fusidate being increased and levels of cephalexin and rifampicin remaining unchanged. It is possible that where increased drug levels have been found they result from decreased metabolism in the gut wall or in the liver.

Altered Gastrointestinal Motility

Because the greater part of drug absorption takes place in the small intestine, slowed gastric emptying and decreased gastrointestinal motility will delay drug absorption. Thus the rate of absorption of paracetamol, lithium, ampicillin, PAS, phenylbutazone, tetracycline and pivampicillin may be expected to be slowed by drugs such as propantheline, the tricyclic antidepressants, antacids, opioids etc. and may be increased by metoclopramide. The amount of drug absorption may be affected when the drug is poorly soluble or where it is formulated as a slow-release or enteric-coated preparation. Thus the absorption of digoxin from some proprietary preparations may be increased by drugs with anticholinergic actions and decreased by metoclopramide or conditions causing gastrointestinal hurry. Corticosteroids and dicoumarol may be similarly affected. L-Dopa is metabolised in gastric mucosa so that rapid gastric emptying tends to increase its bioavailability. Other conditions which tend to cause slowing of gastric emptying include gastric ulcer, pyloric stenosis, migraine, myocardial infarction, trauma and pain.

Table 11.1. Clinically important causes of altered drug absorption/bioavailability

Mechanism	Primary factor	Drug affected	Effect
Reduced mucosal surface	Coeliac disease	Digoxin Penicillin Pivampicillin Thyroxine	Reduced absorption
		Amoxycillin Lincomycin Practolol	Delayed absorption
	Crohn's disease	Lincomycin Metronidazole	Reduced absorption
Increased motility	Acute gastro-intestinal hurry	L-dopa	Increased bioavailability
	Metoclopramide	Corticosteroids Phenytoin Digoxin Dicoumarol Slow-release preparations	Decreased absorption
Decreased motility	Anticholin-ergic drugs Opiates	Digoxin (except Lanoxin) Dicoumarol	Increased absorption
		L-dopa	Decreased bioavailability
pH change	Sodium bicarbonate	Tetracycline L-dopa	Reduced absorption Increased absorption
Binding or chelation	Cholestyramine	Warfarin Thyroxine Digoxin Paracetamol	Reduced absorption
	Calcium Magnesium Aluminium Antacids	Tetracycline	Reduced absorption
	Iron prepara-tions	Tetracycline Sulphasalazine	
Reduced presystemic metabolism	Enzyme-inhib-iting drugs Food Hepatocellular disease Portosystemic shunts Elderly Coeliac disease Crohn's disease	High clearance drugs	Increased bioavailability
Increased presystemic metabolism	Enzyme-inducing drugs	High clearance drugs	Decreased bioavailability

Binding and Chelation of Drugs Within the Gut Lumen

Adsorbents such as kaolin and charcoal and ionic binding agents such as cholestyramine may interfere with the absorption of many drugs. Aluminium-, calcium- and magnesium-containing antacids may combine with tetracycline to form insoluble chelates and, similarly, iron preparations may bind tetracycline.

Effect of Food Intake

Concurrent food intake has been shown to increase the bioavailability of the following drugs either through reduced first pass metabolism or improved tablet dissolution: propranolol, metroprolol, labetalol, hydrallazine, hydrochlorothiazide, nitrofurantoin, carbamazepine, spironolactone, dicoumarol, phenytoin and griseofulvin. Food intake may reduce the bioavailability of the following drugs through altered gastrointestinal motility or pH: isoniazid, L-dopa, penicillins, ampicillin, erythromycin base and rifampicin.

Altered Presystemic Metabolism

A major determinant of bioavailability is the extent of presystemic metabolism in the liver. Only drugs with high hepatic extraction (high clearance agents) will be affected; examples of these drugs are:

Propranolol	Dextropropoxyphene
Metoprolol	Pentazocine
Alprenolol	Nefopam
Labetalol	Nortriptyline
Verapamil	Imipramine
Lignocaine	Chlormethiazole
Glyceryl trinitrate	Metoclopramide
Pethidine	Niridazole
Morphine	

The phenomenon has been little studied but work which has been carried out suggests that there is wide variation between individuals in the activity of the enzymes, so that a two- or threefold difference in drug level after oral administration of these drugs may be expected. Furthermore, enzyme-inducing agents (listed below) may increase the enzyme activity and therefore decrease bioavailability:

Barbiturates	Rifampicin
Glutethimide	Griseofulvin
Dichloralphenazone	Corticosteroids
Phenytoin	Nicotine
Carbamazepine	Ethyl alcohol
Phenylbutazone	Chlorpromazine

Conversely, enzyme-inhibiting drugs (listed below) will increase bioavailability:

Allopurinol	Isoniazid
Chloramphenicol	Metronidazole
Cimetidine	Dextropropoxyphene
Sulthiame	Disulfiram
Sodium valproate	Chlordiazepoxide
Clofibrate	Diazepam
Phenylbutazone	Imipramine
Azapropazone	Perphenazine
Oxyphenbutazone	Procarbazine
Dicoumarol	Chlorpromazine
Sulphaphenazole	Prochlorperazine
Sulphamethizole	
Co-trimoxazole	

Presystemic metabolism is decreased in the elderly, presumably through reduced metabolic capacity, so that bioavailability is increased. In chronic liver disease decreased metabolic capacity and the presence of shunts from portal to systemic circulation cause a marked increase in bioavailability. Particularly care in the oral use of these high clearance agents is indicated where dose adjustment is critical and where these factors are present.

Hepatic Drug Elimination

Drugs which are highly lipid soluble readily cross lipid cell membranes and consequently absorption from the gastrointestinal tract is facilitated. Such drugs tend to penetrate the CNS and indeed most CNS active agents are highly lipid soluble. Lipid soluble agents are not readily excreted by the kidney because as the nephron contents become concentrated the drug merely diffuses back across the tubular epithelium into the blood. In general, lipid-soluble drugs undergo partial or complete biotransformation in the liver to products which are less lipid soluble and more easily excreted by the kidney.

A number of enzyme systems may be involved in the metabolism of a single drug; detailed discussion of these is beyond the scope of this book but two such systems are worthy of mention. *The microsomally located mixed function oxidase system* is important because many drugs are metabolised by these enzymes, which are dependent upon the coenzyme cytochrome P450. Certain drugs and environmental factors may induce increased synthesis of these enzymes and thus increased clearance of other drugs. Drugs may compete for the enzymes and others may inhibit them. The activity of the mixed function oxidase system is largely determined by the interaction of many genes so that there is wide inter-individual difference in the activity of the system. In contrast, the activity of the enzyme *N-acetyl transferase* is governed by a single autosomal dominant gene. There is a bimodal distribution within the population in the rate of metabolism of acetylated drugs, permitting a classification into slow and fast acetylators. The prevalence of the gene varies from country to country; for example the percentage of fast acetylators in Japan is 90%, in Great Britain, 40%, and in Egypt, 18%. In general, slow acetylators are more prone to develop dose related adverse effects of acetylated drugs.

Metabolised drugs may thus be classified according to the enzyme system they use. But they may also be classified into high or low clearance groups according to the avidity with which they are removed from the blood. This classification has important implications when one considers the effect of liver diseases on drug kinetics. In the first place high clearance agents suffer extensive presystemic metabolism. Secondly, the actual clearance rate of highly extracted drugs is more sensitive to changes in hepatic blood flow than to changes in metabolic capacity. It follows that the elimination of such drugs will be changed more obviously by conditions causing haemodynamic derangement. When there is little affinity between enzyme system and drug the elimination rate is insensitive to changes in hepatic blood flow. The elimination half-life of such low clearance drugs is often prolonged in patients with chronic liver disease due to a reduction in the capacity of the hepatic enzyme systems, particularly at the stage of decompensation.

The pharmacokinetics of a large number of drugs in chronic liver disease have not been studied. In early studies workers often failed to demonstrate any effects of liver disease on drug half-life; however, it is now generally accepted that acute and chronic liver disease will cause impairment of clearance of most drugs which are eliminated by the liver. A fall in clearance will result in a similar fall in half-life, assuming no change in distribution volume. Reduction in clearance causes a rise in steady state plasma levels of a drug in the absence of dose changes and prolongation of half-life lengthens the time needed to reach a steady state. It is important to appreciate that the changes in drug kinetics induced by liver disease may actually be smaller than inter-individual variability in the healthy state, so that one cannot predict with certainty the need for dose reduction. Thus demonstration of an effect of liver disease on drug kinetics may be possible when comparing mean values from groups of patients but there may be considerable overlap between results from normal subjects and those from patients with decompensated liver disease. The main effects of chronic liver disease on drug kinetics are:

1. Increased bioavailability—high clearance agents only
2. Reduced clearance—most metabolised drugs
3. Reduced plasma protein binding—certain drugs only
4. Altered tissue distribution—most drugs

The ageing process is accompanied by a progressive deterioration in the activity of drug-metabolising enzyme systems. Many studies have shown that the mean clearance of a number of drugs is significantly lower in groups of elderly people than in young people. However, age accounts for only a small part of the inter-individual variability in drug metabolism and it certainly cannot be presumed that an elderly person will require a reduced dose of a metabolised drug on pharmacokinetic grounds.

Drug Distribution

The physicochemical properties of the individual drug determine the way in which it is transported in the blood and distributed to body organs. Factors such as the water and lipid solubility of the drug and its affinity for certain body proteins as well as the status of regional blood flow determine the final distribution throughout the body. Exact characterisation of drug distribution requires special techniques and is usually carried out in animals. However, a useful measurement in man is the "apparent volume of distribution". This is the volume into which the dose given would have to be diluted to achieve the plasma level. For some drugs the distribution volume actually represents a body compartment; for example, antipyrine is distributed evenly throughout body water and so its distribution volume equates with body water. The apparent distribution volume of those drugs which are taken up and stored in body tissues outside the blood may be many times greater than body volume. For example, digoxin's volume of distribution is about 500 litres. It is important to appreciate that the distribution volume of a drug is one major determinant of drug half-life, the other being clearance, so that

$$\text{Half-life} \propto \frac{\text{Volume of distribution}}{\text{Clearance}}$$

Any variable which alters distribution volume may thus have an effect on drug half-life even if the elimination process remains unchanged. As discussed earlier, the changes in body composition brought about by poor nutrition and by the effect of hepatic disease are important in gastro-enterology. Loss of plasma protein, fluid retention, loss of lean body mass and fat stores all have their influence on drug half-life through influencing distribution volume. The effect on the kinetics of individual agents is difficult to predict and in the absence of studies on each drug the physician must merely be aware that published drug half-lives may be wildly inaccurate with respect to his own patients.

Certain drugs loosely chemically bound to certain plasma proteins, usually albumin or α_1 acid glycoproteins. The protein-bound portion is in equilibrium with the portion which is in solution in the plasma and free to be distributed. Much has been made of drug interactions occurring by one drug displacing another from its binding sites. It has been suggested that certain drugs are potentiated by states in which plasma proteins are depleted; recent evidence suggests that under these circumstances the concentration of drug which is free in the plasma remains unchanged. Total plasma level, which includes the protein bound portion, is reduced. There is, therefore, the risk that if dosage is increased to achieve a certain total plasma level the free drug level will become excessive. Thus the therapeutic range of plasma levels for phenytoin is considerably lower in patients who have altered plasma protein binding; this has been clearly shown in renal failure and is to be expected in the presence of hepatic disease or protein malnutrition.

Tissue Sensitivity

We have seen how disease processes and other variables within the liver and gastrointestinal tract can cause altered drug pharmacokinetics. However, altered drug response and predisposition to adverse drug effects may result from abnormal sensitivity to an appropriate drug concentration. Abnormalities within the body arising from gastrointestinal diseases may give rise to an excessive response to a wide number of different types of drug. For example, where fluid and electrolyte depletion has occurred, concurrent administration of diuretic drugs might precipitate profound hypokalaemia and prerenal uraemia and concurrent administration of antihypertensive drugs might produce an excessive fall in blood pressure. Patients with malnutrition may be particularly sensitive to the adverse effects of corticosteroids, while those with potential bleeding sources such as peptic ulceration or ulcerative colitis may be particularly sensitive to the non-steroidal anti-inflammatory agents and oral anticoagulants. For this reason it is important that the physician faced with an acute or chronic gastrointestinal problem should review the drugs being prescribed for other conditions, perhaps by other doctors, and should bear in mind the effects that each drug is having on the patient and the interaction between drugs and disease processes. In complicated cases it may be necessary to give priority to one aspect of the case over another. Undoubtedly patients with severe liver disease are those most at risk of developing adverse drug effects, both because of the marked effect of liver disease on pharmacokinetics described above and because these patients are highly susceptible to precipitation of hepatic encephalopathy by a number of different mechanisms. Thus any drug causing electrolyte abnormalities is at risk of precipitating encephalopathy. Any drug slowing gastrointestinal motility may increase bacterial breakdown of protein within the gut, and these patients are highly susceptible to modest doses of CNS depressants. In conclusion, therefore, Table 11.2 lists the special precautions required in prescribing drugs for patients with severe liver disease.

Table 11.2. Drugs requiring special precautions in severe liver disease

Drug	Effect	Reason	Recommendation
Phenothiazines Tetracyclic antidepressants Chlormethiazide	Excessive sedation or precipitation of encephalopathy	Increased bioavailability Reduced clearance Altered distribution Increased CNS sensitivity	Avoid
Butyrophenones Benzodiazepines Anticonvulsants Antihistamines	Excessive sedation or precipitation of encephalopathy	Altered distribution Reduced clearance Increased CNS sensitivity	Avoid
Opiates and Opioids	Precipitation of encephalopathy	Increased bioavailability Reduced clearance	Avoid
Tricyclic antidepressants	Precipitation of encephalopathy	Increased CNS sensitivity Reduced gastrointestinal motility	Avoid
Anticholinergics, e.g. disopyramide, orphenadrine, propantheline	Precipitation of encephalopathy	Reduced gastrointestinal motility	Monitor CNS function
Diuretics	Precipitation of encephalopathy	Hypokalaemia Hyponatraemia Volume depletion	Slow diuresis Use amiloride (low potency, potassium sparing)
Spironolactone	Exacerbation of gynaecomastia	Oestrogen-like	Use amiloride or triamterene
Corticosteroids Cortisone Prednisone	Increased adverse effects Reduced effect	Reduced clearance Failure to convert to active moiety	Monitor drug carefully Use cortisol or prednisolone
Carbenoxolone	Precipitation of fluid retention Precipitation of encephalopathy	Increased sensitivity to adverse effects	Avoid
Cimetidine	Confusional states more common May exacerbate condition	Reduce liver blood flow	Monitor effect carefully

Table 11.2. *(continued)*

Drug	Effect	Reason	Recommendation
Propranolol Labetalol Metoprolol	Excessive effect	Increased bioavailability	Monitor effect carefully
Lignocaine Theophylline Verapamil	Cardiotoxicity Increased toxicity Excessive effect likely	Markedly reduced clearance Reduced clearance Increased bioavailability likely	Avoid or monitor blood level Avoid or monitor blood level Exercise caution
Anticoagulants	Bleeding	Increased sensitivity Decreased clearance	Check prothrombin time before starting Use reduced dose Monitor daily initially
Metoclopramide Antacids containing sodium Antacids containing calcium	Increased adverse effects Fluid retention Precipitation of encephalopathy	Increased bioavailability Unable to correct sodium load Decreased gastrointestinal motility	Adjust dose Avoid Avoid

Cholestyramine
Non-steroidal anti-
   inflammatory
	Prolongation of prothrombin time
	Increased incidence of
	   gastrointestinal bleeding
	Fluid retention
		Causes vitamin K malabsorption
		Increased sensitivity
			Monitor effect
			Avoid if possible

Paracetamol	Exacerbation of liver disease	Direct hepatotoxicity	Avoid large doses or prolonged treatment
Monoamine oxidase inhibitors	Exacerbation of liver disease	High incidence of idiosyncratic hepatotoxicity	Avoid
Biguanides	Excessive hypoglycaemia Risk of lactic acidosis	Increased sensitivity Decreased elimination	Avoid
Sulphonylureas	Excessive hypoglycaemia Exacerbation of liver disease	Increased sensitivity Decreased clearance Cholestatic jaundice	Avoid

Table 11.2. (continued)

Drug	Effect	Reason	Recommendation
Methotrexate	Exacerbation of liver disease	Direct hepatotoxicity	Avoid
Oral contraceptives	Exacerbation of liver disease	Increased risk of cholestatic jaundice	Avoid in patients with history of cholestasis in pregnancy
Vitamin D	Reduced effect	Failure to convert to active moiety	Use 1,25-dihydroxycholecalciferol or 1α-hydroxycholecalciferol
Chloramphenicol	Risk of bone marrow depression	Decreased clearance	Avoid
Clindamycin	Increased toxicity	Decreased clearance	Reduced dose
Fusidic acid	Increased toxicity, especially hepatic	Decreased biliary elimination	Avoid or reduce dose
Isoniazid Pyrazinamide	Increased toxicity	Decreased clearance	Avoid
Rifampicin	Risk of hepatotoxicity	Decreased clearance	Avoid or reduce dose
Niridazole	CNS toxicity	Increased bioavailability	Reduce dose
Tetracycline	Exacerbation of liver disease	Direct hepatotoxicity at high dose	Avoid i.v. route of administration
Talampicillin	Exacerbation of liver disease	Unhydrolysed dry hepatotoxic	Avoid
Suxamethonium	Prolonged neuromuscular blockade	Decreased levels of pseudocholinesterase	Caution
Erythromycin estolate	Exacerbation of liver disease	Hepatotoxicity	Avoid
Sulphonamides	Increased toxic effects possible	Decreased hepatic clearance	Use alternative therapy or monitor effect carefully
Chloroquine Pyrimethamine	Increased toxic effects	Decreased clearance	Avoid
Thiabendazole	Increased toxic effects	Decreased clearance	Reduce dose
Allopurinol	Increased toxicity	Reduced clearance	Reduce dose

Further Reading

Black M (1974) Liver disease and drug therapy. Med Clin North Am 58(5): 1051–1057

Blaschke TF (1977) Protein binding and kinetics of drugs in liver disease. Clinical Pharmacokinetics 2: 32–44

Blaschke TF, Rubin PC (1979) Hepatic first pass metabolism in liver disease. Clinical Pharmacokinetics 4: 423–432

Farrell GC et al. (1978) Drug metabolism in liver disease. Identification of patients with impaired hepatic drug metabolism. Gastroenterology 75: 580–588

George CF (1979) Drug kinetics and hepatic blood flow. Clinical Pharmacokinetics 4: 433–448

George CF (1981) Drug metabolism by the gastrointestinal mucosa. Clinical Pharmacokinetics 6: 259–274

Gugler R et al. (1975) Effect of portacaval shunt on the disposition of drugs with and without first pass effect. J Pharmacol Exp Ther 195: 416–423

Hurwitz A (1977) Antacid therapy and drug kinetics. Clinical Pharmacokinetics 2: 269–280

James I (1975) Prescribing in patients with liver disease. Br J Hosp Med 13: 67–76

Levine RR (1970) Factors affecting gastrointestinal absorption of drugs. Am J Digestive Diseases 15: 171–188

Melander A (1979) Influence of food on the bioavailability of drugs. Clinical Pharmacokinetics 3: 337–351

Nies AS et al. (1976) Altered hepatic blood flow and drug disposition. Clinical Pharmacokinetics 1: 135–155

Nimmo WS (1976) Drugs, diseases and altered gastric emptying. Clinical Pharmacokinetics 1: 189

Park BK, Breckenridge AM (1981) Clinical implications of enzyme induction and enzyme inhibition. Clinical Pharmacokinetics 6: 1–24

Parsons RL (1977) Drug absorption in gastrointestinal disease with particular reference to malabsorption syndromes. Clinical Pharmacokinetics 2: 45–60

Prescott LF (1974) Gastrointestinal absorption of drugs. Med Clin North Am 58(5): 907–916

Roberts RK et al. (1979) Drug prescribing in hepato-biliary disease. Drugs 17: 198–212

Wilkinson GR, Schenker S (1976) Effect of liver disease on drug disposition in man. Biochem Pharmacol 25: 2675–2681

Williams RL, Mamelok RD (1980) Hepatic disease and drug pharmacokinetics. Clinical Pharmacokinetics 5: 528–547

12 Drug Toxicity in the Gastrointestinal Tract and Liver

C. J. C. Roberts

Introduction

Drug toxicity manifests itself frequently within the gastrointestinal tract. The toxic reactions may be trivial and transient, such as the gastrointestinal upset sometimes experienced at the initiation of metformin therapy. There can be few drugs which have not been blamed by patients for causing indigestion, anorexia, constipation or diarrhoea. However, serious or life-threatening iatrogenic disease is also to be found within the gastrointestinal tract in the form of drug-induced peptic ulceration and antibiotic-induced colitis. It would not be possible in this section to cover such reactions comprehensively. The aim here is to remind the physician of those drugs which are commonly responsible for patients presenting with gastrointestinal symptoms. A careful drug history can save much in time, expense and patient discomfort.

Nausea and Vomiting

Anorexia, nausea and vomiting may indicate the presence of disease of the gastrointestinal tract but these symptoms are commonly the presenting features of systemic illness or metabolic abnormality. The gastroenterologist must be aware that patients presenting with these symptoms may be suffering from a systemic adverse drug effect or from a more specific drug-induced gastrointestinal lesion. The author has seen a patient in whom barium meal examinations were performed for symptoms attributable to diuretic-induced hyponatraemia in one case and vitamin D-induced hypercalcaemia in another. All drug therapy should arouse suspicion as a factor in this non-specific complaint. A high incidence of nausea is associated with certain drugs and for many of these the side-effect is consistently dose related. Some drugs induce nausea centrally by stimulating the chemoreceptor trigger zone in the floor of the fourth ventricle (central action) while others have an irritant effect on the mucosa of the stomach or small intestine (local action). Some examples are listed in Table 12.1.

Table 12.1. Drugs inducing nausea and vomiting

Centrally acting	Locally acting	Unclassified
Digoxin	Theophylline	Dapsone
L-dopa	Erythromycin	Clofibrate
Opiates	Iron salts	Spironolactone
Oestrogens	Metformin	
Oncolytics	Penicillamine	
Theophylline	Potassium chloride	
Gold salts	Quinidine	
Lithium	Reserpine	
Nitrofurantoin	Tetracycline	
Sulphonamides	Cephalosporins	
Fenfluramine	Chloral hydrate	
Diethylpropion	Cholestyramine	
Isoxsuprine	Non-steroidal anti-inflammatory agents	
Mexiletine		
Sulphasalazine		

Diarrhoea and Constipation

Diarrhoea may be part of a non-specific drug-induced gastrointestinal upset or may be brought about by specific mechanisms within the gut (Table 12.2). Antacids containing magnesium salts tend to increase the faecal water content

Table 12.2. Examples of drug-induced diarrhoea

Mechanism	Drug group
Osmotic loading	Magnesium-containing antacids
	Bulking agents
Nerve plexus stimulation	Anthraquinones
Altered gut bacteria	Antibiotics
Sympathetic nervous blockade	Adrenergic neurone blocking agents
Malabsorption syndrome	Neomycin
	Cholestyramine
Bile salt load	Chenodeoxycholic acid
Non-specific gastrointestinal upset	Digoxin
	Anti-inflammatory agents
	Gold salts and penicillamine

by their osmotic effect and thus cause diarrhoea. Conversely, aluminium and calcium salts tend to harden the faeces and render them less easily propelled by peristaltic waves and therefore cause constipation. Drugs may interfere with the autonomic control of gut. Gut mobility is stimulated by the parasympathetic nervous system and inhibited by the sympathetic. Thus drugs with an anticholinergic action will tend to cause constipation whilst sympatholytics predispose to diarrhoea.

Other examples of groups of drugs liable to cause constipation are given in Table 12.3. These drugs should be avoided in patients with a tendency to constipation, especially the elderly, as there is a real risk of their causing faecal impactions.

Table 12.3. Some examples of drug-induced constipation

Mechanism	Drug group
Reduced peristalsis Increased smooth muscle tone	All opiates and synthetic analogues
Parasympathetic blockade	Tricyclic antidepressants Anti-parkinsonian drugs Phenothiazines Disopyramide
Sedation	Benzodiazepines Antihistamines etc.
Altered faecal sensitivity	Aluminium- and calcium-containing antacids Ferrous sulphate Barium sulphate Calcium resonium

Some of the more important drug-induced diarrhoeal syndromes are considered below.

Antibiotic-Associated Colitis

Almost all antibiotics have at some time been incriminated in causing severe diarrhoea or colitis. The exact cause remains in dispute but attention has focused in recent years on the high incidence of toxin from *Clostridium difficile* in the faeces of such patients. It has been postulated that antibiotic therapy predisposes to the growth of this organism, which is the common factor in the production of antibiotic colitis. The spectrum of severity of the condition is wide. It may carry a mortality of 70% in patients over 65 years of age, so that early diagnosis and correct treatment are mandatory.

Diagnosis

Patients present with diarrhoea (with or without blood), abdominal pain, cramps and fever, and occasionally with severe toxicity and shock. Colitis may develop after exposure to one of the following antibiotics:

Common: Lincomycin, clindamycin, ampicillin

Uncommon: Tetracycline, penicillin, co-trimoxazole, cephalosporins, chloramphenicol, metronidazole

Antibiotic-associated colitis is particularly liable to occur in the elderly and immobile, in chronic laxative abusers, and in those who have been treated with constipating agents. All these factors favour the proliferation of *Clostridium difficile*.

Proctosigmoidoscopy reveals inflamed and ulcerated rectal mucosa and sometimes the presence of a pseudomembrane due to plaques of exudate.

Where antibiotic-associated colitis is strongly suspected, treatment should not be delayed and stool should be tested for the presence of *Clostridium difficile* toxin. Rectal biopsy reveals characteristic histological appearance of leucocyte infiltration of lamina propria, necrosis and purulent pseudomembranes.

Treatment

Vancomycin 1–2 g daily in divided doses or metronidazole 400 mg 8 hourly for 5 days should be administered orally. Topical or systemic steroids may be required, particularly when toxic megacolon occurs.

Prevention of Cross Infection

Nurse patients with precautions similar to those adopted for enteric fevers. Sigmoidoscopes etc. should be sterilised with an effective germicidal agent such as glutaraldehyde.

Laxative Abuse

Vast amounts of laxatives are bought and consumed by the populus. Such consumption is largely unnecessary and results from inadequate education, custom and poor diet. The appropriate use of laxatives is restricted to short courses in patients in whom acute constipation with discomfort has developed, in patients in whom straining at stool might be hazardous, e.g. following anal

surgery, myocardial infarction and intracranial haemorrhage, and in preparation for gastrointestinal investigation or procedures. Occasionally patients
suffer adverse effects from habitual laxative use. When taken over many years
and in high dosage, irritant laxatives, particularly anthraquinones, may cause
damage to the myenteric plexus and alteration of large bowel function with
atony and loss of haustrations. Smooth contractions of the bowel (pseudostric-
tures) may be seen radiographically. Sigmoidoscopic examination differenti-
ates the condition from ulcerative colitis and may reveal the presence of
pigmentation in the mucosa due to lipofuscin-containing macrophages. If the
patient can be persuaded to stop the laxative, normal function and appearances
may return during the following months. Apart from the damaging effect of
chronic laxatives on the bowel, the chronic diarrhoea may lead to deficiencies
of potassium, resulting in weakness, nephropathy and cardiac abnormalities,
and of magnesium and calcium. Abnormal xylose absorption and protein-
losing enteropathy also occur and it is likely that the absorption of many drugs
will be abnormal in the presence of laxative use. Occasionally manipulative
patients are encountered who induce diarrhoea in themselves following the use
of purgatives. Examination for phenolphthalein in the faeces by alkalination or
other methods of detection may be required.

Malabsorption Syndromes

Although a number of drugs are implicated in causing specific deficiencies by
one mechanism or another, a malabsorption syndrome with steatorrhoea and
multiple deficiencies is rarely attributable to drug treatment. Cytotoxic drugs
and colchicine may cause damage to small intestinal mucosa, leading to partial
villous atrophy and a syndrome similar to coeliac disease. Neomycin,
tetracyclines and para-aminosalicylic acid can also cause widespread malabsorption by altering normal gut bacteria. Cholestyramine can induce
steatorrhoea and fat-soluble vitamin deficiencies by binding bile salts within
the gut lumen.

Mucosal Ulceration and Bleeding

Damage to the epithelium of the upper gastrointestinal tract is a common
adverse drug effect. Mucosal ulceration or bleeding may occur as a direct
chemical effect of the drug in contact with the mucosa or it may be a
consequence of some systemic effect of the drug which predisposes to the
development of peptic ulceration. Thus emepronium bromide and slow-
release potassium preparations are implicated in causing oesophageal
ulceration if allowed to remain in contact with oesophageal mucosa for a

prolonged period. Special care has to be taken in prescribing these drugs in patients with poor oesophageal motility as might occur in the presence of hiatus hernia, oesophageal stricture, the elderly or patients with cardiomegaly. In such patients it is advisable to use a soluble potassium preparation and the tablets should be taken with a drink and with the patient sitting in the upright position. Patients at risk should not take these preparations last thing at night. It should be remembered that a similar effect in the small intestine was seen after use of enteric-coated potassium preparations. These preparations have now been withdrawn in the United Kingdom because of the ulceration and the small bowel stricture formation which they caused.

Aspirin is well-known to have a direct damaging effect on gastric mucosa, causing a rise in faecal occult blood loss in all individuals. Although most physicians will have seen patients presenting with massive gastrointestinal haemorrhage after the acute ingestion of aspirin tablets and iron deficiency anaemia in the chronic aspirin user, the epidemiologist would regard these associations as far from proven. The reason is that some studies have failed to show a clear relationship between aspirin and gastrointestinal haemorrhage although other non-steroidal anti-inflammatory agents have been clearly implicated. Despite the controversy, most physicians would regard aspirin and all non-steroidal anti-inflammatory agents as potentially hazardous in the gastrointestinal tract. In the presence of peptic ulceration it seems that aspirin and other non-steroidal anti-inflammatory agents are implicated in causing perforation.

Whether or not certain groups of drugs actually predispose to the development of peptic ulcers also remains controversial. One might expect the anti-inflammatory and protein-catabolising effect of corticosteroids to prevent the healing of superficial ulceration and to allow the development of large gastric ulcers with little symptomatology. Cytotoxic and immunosuppressant drugs may slow epithelial cell turnover and break down the gastric mucosal barrier. Non-steroidal anti-inflammatory agents also appear to break down gastromucosal barriers, possibly by suppressing gastric mucus production, but the exact role of these drugs in the aetiology of peptic ulcer disease is controversial. Regular ingestion of aspirin in women has been shown to predispose to the development of gastric ulceration, but with other anti-inflammatory agents this relationship is not proven. Whilst most physicians will have seen patients with large shallow gastric ulcers, in patients with rheumatoid arthritis on long-term steroid therapy it is not yet clear whether these ulcers relate more closely to the therapy or to the disease process itself. Clearly, very large doses of systemic steroids equivalent to 1 g prednisolone can produce gastric ulcers. The situation is further complicated by the fact that many patients complain of dyspepsia symptoms when receiving corticosteroids or anti-inflammatory agents without any demonstrable lesion of the gastrointestinal tract. Such symptoms can be partially prevented by the use of enteric-coated preparations, suppositories and pro-drugs. Finally it should be appreciated that rectal ulceration is occasionally drug induced, when certain drugs are administered by suppository. Indomethacin, bisacodyl and aminophylline may all cause proctitis and occasionally superficial ulceration.

Drug-Induced Pancreatic Disease

A number of drugs have been implicated in causing acute pancreatitis. No other pancreatic lesion has a drug-induced aetiology. There are, of course, problems in the interpretation of a myriad of case reports which vary widely in the standard of documentation. Rarely have the patients suffering pancreatitis been rechallenged with the suspected drug; indeed, such rechallenge would be highly questionable ethically in the majority of cases. Table 12.4 outlines the groups of drugs strongly suspected of causing pancreatitis; knowledge of these drugs enables the physician faced with a case of pancreatitis to examine the recent drug history and warn that future exposure to a suspected agent should be avoided.

Table 12.4. Suspected drug-induced pancreatitis

Drug	Weight of evidence
Asparaginase	Poor
Azathioprine	Many case reports but often concomitant corticosteroids
Calcium+vitamin D	Only in presence of hypercalcaemia
Cimetidine	One case report. Some experimental work in rats. Unlikely cause
Clofibrate	Causes gall-stones and subsequent pancreatitis
Corticosteroids	Probably implicated. Many case reports
Diazoxide	Possible
Diuretics	Many case reports with various diuretics and some controlled surveys of cases of pancreatitis. Probably implicated
Methyldopa	Single case report with rechallenge Probably implicated
Oestrogens	Several case reports. Some cases in association with type V hyperlipidaemia
Pentamidine	Possible
Phenformin	Several case reports but definite association not proven
Procainamide	Single case report with rechallenge
Rifampicin	Reports of raised serum amylase only
Sulindac	Two reports, one with rechallenge
Sulphasalazine	Single case report with rechallenge
Tetracycline	Pancreatitis accompanies acute fatty liver of pregnancy, which may be precipitated by tetracycline
Valproic acid	Several case reports, one with rechallenge

Drug-Induced Liver Disease

The liver is the organ of the body most susceptible to adverse drug effects. This is because high concentrations are presented to the liver after absorption from the gastrointestinal tract and toxic metabolites may be formed within the liver.

Table 12.5. Drug-induced hepatic disease

Predominant lesion	Predictability	Drugs
Hepatitis-like	Predictable	Paracetamol
Hepatitis-like	Unpredictable	Halothane, monoamine oxidase inhibitors, sulphonamides, phenytoin, pyrazinamide, ethionamide, isoniazid, methyldopa, sodium valproate, carbamazepine, lincomycin
Cholestasis	Predictable	C_{17}-substituted steroids (methyltestosterone and norethandrolone)
	Unpredictable	Erythromycin estolate, chlorpromazine and other phenothiazines, oral contraceptives, azathioprine, penicillamine, fusidicaciel
Mixed features (cholestatic hepatitis)	Unpredictable	Rifampicin (increased susceptibility in slow acetylators and those taking isoniazid), para-aminosalicylic acid, propyl thiouracil, imipramine, nitrofurantoin
Granulomatous hepatitis	Unpredictable	Hydrallazine, phenylbutazone
Fatty liver of pregnancy	Predictable	Tetracyline (large intravenous doses in 1st trimester of pregnancy)
Cirrhosis	Predictable (prolonged regular treatment)	Methotrexate, paracetamol
Hepatic adenomata and focal nodular hyperplasia	?	Oral contraceptives
Chronic active hepatitis	Unpredictable	Methyldopa, oxyphenisatin, isoniazid, aspirin

Many drugs are abandoned during development because of alterations in liver function tests or the appearance of frank hepatotoxicity. Even so, a myriad of drugs capable of producing hepatic reactions of one type or another are available to the prescriber. So common a problem is drug-induced jaundice that any patient presenting with jaundice requires careful scrutiny of their immediate past drug history. Classification of the types of hepatotoxicity due to drugs is difficult because many of the mechanisms involved are poorly understood. Although it is possible to talk of hepatocellular jaundice and cholestatic jaundice, in practice patients will have a mixture of features. Certain drugs may cause a transient rise in liver enzymes which is generally regarded as being of no consequence. In classifying drug hepatotoxicity it is important to distinguish between predictable and unpredictable reactions. Direct hepatotoxins are drugs or substances for which one can predict a hepatic reaction in 100% of cases if the dose is high enough. The single most important example of this type of hepatotoxicity is that due to paracetamol. The more common type of hepatotoxicity is an unpredictable reaction to a drug unrelated to the dose taken and representing an idiosyncratic reaction to the drug on the part of the patient. Drug reactions may be predominantly hepatocellular or predominantly cholestatic, or chronic changes may appear, such as cirrhosis or granulomata. The main purpose of Table 12.5 is to provide a workable classification of drug hepatotoxicity together with examples. It would not be possible to provide a comprehensive list of all known drug reactions in this text, and the reader is referred to *Meyler's Side Effects of Drugs* for a comprehensive review. Other aspects of the management of drug-induced liver disease are presented in Chap. 8.

Further Reading

Bell GD (1980) Drugs used in the management of gallstones. In: Dukes MNG (ed) Meyler's side effects of drugs, 9th edn. Excerpta Medica, Amsterdam Oxford Princeton, p 626

Bell GD (1980) Drugs used in the management of gallstones. In: Dukes MNG (ed) Side effects of drugs, annual 4. Excerpta Medica, Amsterdam Oxford Princeton, p 258

Benson JA (1971) Gastrointestinal reactions to drugs. Am J Dig Dis 16: 357–362

Bourke JB et al. (1978) Drug associated primary acute pancreatitis. Lancet I: 706–708

Bramble MG, Record CO (1978) Drug induced gastrointestinal disease. Drugs 15: 451–463

Cameron AJ (1975) Aspirin and gastric ulcer. Mayo Clin Proc 50: 565–570

Cooke AR (1976) Drugs and gastric damage. Drugs 11: 36–44

Cuthbert MF (1974) Adverse reactions to non-steroidal anti-rheumatic drugs. Curr Med Res Opin 2: 600–609

Douglas AP, Bateman DN (1981) Gastrointestinal disorders. In: Davies DM (ed) Textbook of adverse drug reactions, 2nd edn. Oxford Univ Press, Oxford New York Toronto p 202

Editorial (1975) Antibiotic diarrhoea. Br Med J 4: 243–244

Gallagher ND, Goulston SJM (1978) Antibiotic associated colitis. In search of a cause and treatment. Drugs 16: 385–386

Jick H, Porter J (1978) Drug induced gastrointestinal bleeding. Report from the Boston Collaborative Drug Surveillance Program. Boston University Medical Centre. Lancet II: 87–89

Langman MJS (1980) Gastrointestinal drugs. In: Dukes MNG (ed) Meyler's side effects of drugs, 9th edn. Excerpta Medica, Amsterdam Oxford Princeton, p 618

Langman MJS (1980) Gastrointestinal drugs. In: Dukes MNG (ed) Side effects of drugs, annual 4. Excerpta Medica, Amsterdam Oxford Princeton, p 252

Langstreth GF, Newcome AD (1975) Drug induced malabsorption. Mayo Clin Proc 50: 284–293

Lendrum R (1981) Drugs and the pancreas. Adverse Drug Reaction Bulletin 90: 328–331

Maxwell JD, Williams R (1971) Adverse drug reactions and the liver. Adverse Drug Reaction Bulletin 29: 84–87

Sherlock S (1969) Factors determining hepatic reactions to drugs. Ann NY Acad Sci 160: 775–782

Sladen GE (1972) Effects of chronic purgative abuse. Proc R Soc Med 65: 288–291

Smith ER, Goulston SJM (1974) Antibiotic induced diarrhoea. Drugs 10: 329–332

Stewart RB, Cluff LE (1974) Gastrointestinal manifestation of adverse drug reactions. Am J Dig Dis 19: 1–7

Zimmerman HJ (1978) Drug induced liver disease. Drugs 16: 25–45

13 Nutritional Support in Gastrointestinal Disease

M. J. Hall

Introduction

An adequate and balanced supply of nutrients and energy is necessary for maintenance of a normal nutritional state. The concept of an ideal weight recognises the morbidity and mortality associated with under- or over-nutrition. Increasing awareness of the importance of nutrition in health and disease has resulted in a formidable expansion of the number of commercially manufactured nutritional preparations. It is important that clear principles should be established for the choice and the use of these products. An appreciation of the prevalence of nutritional deficiency, of its causes and of its potential consequences is fundamental to assessing nutritional status and providing nutritional support. Consideration must be given to the method to be employed—whether it is to be oral, enteral or parenteral, and whether it is to be supplemental to an ordinary oral diet or instead of it. The regime chosen must be nutritionally balanced and tailored to the clinical requirements. If certain guidelines are followed the provision of enteral or parenteral nutrition is a safe procedure, but monitoring of clinical and biochemical parameters is essential. Before embarking on a nutritional support programme, the aims of the treatment must be defined. Regular anthropometric measurements and other forms of nutritional assessment will provide an indication of progress and can be a source of encouragement to both patient and physician.

Prevalence of Nutritional Deficiency

Surveys in hospitals have shown clinical, biochemical and immunological evidence of malnutrition in many medical and surgical patients independent of underlying disease.

Gastrointestinal and related problems are frequently associated with poor nutritional status. The significance of anorexia is often underestimated, so that the unattractive presentation of institutionally prepared food may fail to stimulate the appetite of many hospital patients. Poor intake may develop through fear of associated pain in some cases of peptic ulcer or Crohn's disease. Dysphagia from a simple stricture or oesophageal carcinoma and prolonged vomiting, especially in association with pyloric stenosis, will rapidly result in weight loss. Pancreatic and biliary tract disease may lead to maldigestion and resulting malabsorption. Crohn's disease may be complicated by internal fistulae, blind loops with bacterial overgrowth and chronic discharging external fistulae, leading to malabsorption and subsequent weight loss. Repeated intestinal resection in Crohn's disease or total resection of a gangrenous small bowel after a mesenteric vascular occlusion may produce a "short bowel syndrome" where there is simply insufficient gut to absorb adequate nutrients.

Gastrointestinal surgery may be complicated by nutritional deficiency. The underlying pathology, the catabolic response to the operation itself and prolongation of the normal postoperative ileus are all potential contributory factors. A highly catabolic state is well recognised after trauma or severe burns. It also complicates serious illness such as fulminant ulcerative colitis. In these circumstances catabolism of body proteins exceeds anabolism and the normal dietary protein intake is unable to redress the balance. Features include a negative nitrogen and potassium balance, retention of sodium and water and the accumulation of acid leading to muscle wasting, hypoproteinaemic oedema, apathy and increased susceptibility to infection. Any patient who loses more than 30% of his initial body weight in an acute illness has a poor chance of survival, but early intervention and nutritional support can prevent this.

Liver disease is frequently complicated by significant protein energy malnutrition, but a normal body weight due to fluid retention may mask its presence unless alternative measurements are made. In hepatic encephalopathy many patients are deprived of protein altogether or are given only limited amounts. Because of the danger of precipitating hepatic coma, standard nutritional support cannot be used and this special problem is considered towards the end of the chapter.

Consequences of Protein Energy Malnutrition

It is not difficult to appreciate that severe protein energy malnutrition is a pathological state. The patient appears apathetic and emaciated with a lax wrinkled skin. Marked muscle weakness with inability to stand, dry falling hair and dependent oedema are characteristic, with additional features of anaemia or a specific vitamin deficiency.

Happily this description applies only to a small number of patients. Less obvious nutritional deficiency may still be associated with a depression of cell-mediated immunological competence, leading to increased susceptibility to infections. Immunological anergy on skin testing with commonly encountered antigens has been widely demonstrated and refeeding can correct this.

It has, however, been demonstrated convincingly that wound infection is reduced postoperatively if pre-operative feeding is undertaken, and length of stay in hospital can also be reduced.

Assessment of Nutritional Status

As the nutritional status of an individual is a function of intake, utilisation and possible excretion of a large number of essential nutrients, no single criterion of nutritional deficiency can be laid down. The following is a list of some of the parameters in widespread use (for reference values, see Blackburn and Kaminski 1980) and a combination of anthropometric, biochemical and immunological tests should be performed for an accurate assessment, both in identification of malnutrition and monitoring progress of nutritional support.

Weight (% ideal)
Weight loss
Triceps skinfold thickness
Arm muscle circumference
Creatinine height index
Serum albumin
Serum transferrin
Serum retinol binding protein
Lymphocyte count
Cell mediated immunity to:
   Candida albicans
   Mumps
   PPD (tuberculin)
   Streptokinase/streptodornase
   Trichophyton

Weight as a percentage of ideal weight for height and sex, obtained from established tables, is a reasonable overall reflection of somatic status in many patients. A recent weight loss of more than 15% is associated with increased morbidity, and most authorities take a weight loss of 10% or more as an indication for nutritional support. Reliance should not be placed on simple body weight as oedema may mask nutritional depletion.

Measurement of the triceps skinfold thickness using calipers and expressed as a percentage of ideal for sex is a reflection of body fat stores. Calculation of the arm muscle circumference from the arm circumference by the formula

$$\text{arm muscle circumference} = \text{arm circumference} - (\pi \times \text{triceps skinfold thickness})$$

assumes that the arm is circular and that fat deposition is uniform, but good correlation with muscle bulk has been shown from CT scan measurements. Both measurements should be taken at the mid-point of the non-dominant upper arm, and if serial observations are to be performed they should be carried out by the same operator. The creatinine height index, the percentage of ideal creatinine excretion for height, is said to be an accurate reflection of muscle mass although there is not universal agreement about its usefulness.

Serum albumin and, more recently, transferrin and retinol binding protein are used as a reflection of visceral protein status but recovery of serum proteins does not seem to parallel the nutritional improvements indicated by anthropometric measurements.

Immunological parameters include the absolute lymphocyte count and skin testing with common antigens. This latter test is a sensitive indicator of the ability to mount a cell-mediated response and is simple to perform. The test assumes the antigens used have been met before and to reduce error it is recommended that a battery of five antigens are used, with anergy being defined as a positive response (induration greater than 5 mm) to less than two. In practice the use of *Candida albicans* antigen would give reasonable results in most patients.

The advantages of these tests is that they can be performed rapidly and are within the capability of most laboratories. More complex investigations of total body composition have been developed but these are confined to research centres and have no place in clinical practice. They include the calculation of total body potassium as a reflection of lean body mass by measurement of the naturally occurring isotope of potassium, ^{40}K, using a whole body monitor, neutron activation analysis to measure total body nitrogen and tritiated water dilution to measure total body water.

Urinary 3-methylhistidine derived mainly from muscle is gaining in popularity as a reflection of the degree of muscle breakdown.

Indications for Nutritional Support

The techniques outlined in the previous paragraphs enable a reasonable assessment of the nutritional status of a patient to be made. However, identifying a deficit is not in itself sufficient indication for embarking on a comprehensive regimen of nutritional support. In developed nations it is unlikely that many patients will not have had access to a normal diet although some elderly people will be neglectful of themselves and have poor dietary habits. In the majority, some other factor can be incriminated.

Anorexia, secondary to physical and psychological factors, is difficult to overcome with an oral diet, however attractively it is presented or however frequently the patient is persuaded to take nutritional beverages. The blunt but succinct comment that "anorexia stops at the mouth" reflects the good response that such patients make if higher centres are bypassed and an enteral tube is passed. In many patients anorexia is secondary to the malnutrition itself, and frequently correction of the nutritional deficiency abolishes the anorexia and a normal diet can be resumed.

When surgery is indicated in conditions such as oesophageal carcinoma or gastric outlet obstruction, decisions will be weighted by the degree of urgency of the operation against the benefit obtained by feeding the patient. Neurological problems of oesophageal function may be transient, but it may be impossible to assess how long feeding will be required and long-term administration continued at home may have to be considered. This latter approach is necessary after extensive small bowel resection, where recovery by intestinal adaptation may be expected but not guaranteed.

Where malnutrition has arisen from some systemic disease, particularly inflammatory bowel disease, one should consider how quickly control of the disease activity is likely to be achieved and allow gain in weight by normal diet. Many clinicians feel that giving nutritional support in these circumstances is in fact "buying more than time", and that correction of a nutritional deficit itself will lead to a quicker resolution of the disease process. Whether bowel rest results in a resolution of inflammatory bowel disease is controversial and unproven and is considered in a little more detail below.

Finally, even if the causative factors have resolved, the degree of protein energy malnutrition itself may be an indication for nutritional support in order to achieve weight gain and nutritional recovery more quickly than would be the case with resumption of a normal diet. Patients in this category have little or no fat stores, with triceps skinfold thicknesses between 2 and 5 mm, and are usually less than 60% of their ideal weight.

Prevention rather than correction of nutritional deficiency may be indicated in neurological cases, where the inability to swallow may occur acutely and where full recovery can often be expected. The postoperative period often carries the risk of starvation if appropriate measures are not taken.

In catabolic states feeding should be instituted to prevent malnutrition rather than waiting for it to occur. Many patients in this category, such as those with multiple trauma or burns, will be unable to take food orally and those whose gastrointestinal tract is accessible and functional may not be able to cope with the gross negative nitrogen balance which occurs by sole reliance on the oral route.

Selection of Method of Nutrition

Once the decision to provide the patient with nutritional support has been taken, the route of administration must be selected. The gastrointestinal tract can be utilised, or direct access to the venous system sought via a peripheral or central vein. Theoretically, provided there is no obstruction of access, either anorexic, neurological or mechanical, to a functioning gastrointestinal tract, the oral route can be used. In practice the nursing time required for supervision of intake and the unpalatability of drinking large quantities of flavoured liquid diets make the oral route unsatisfactory in all but the mildest cases.

In most cases the choice lies between an enterally placed tube and the intravenous route. Many previously accepted indications for parenteral nutrition now need to be challenged and to enable the correct route to be selected a number of questions must be asked.

1. *Is the gastrointestinal tract accessible?*
Most oesophageal carcinomas do not obstruct the lumen entirely, and modern techniques will usually allow the passage of a catheter. If the need for nutritional support postoperatively is predicted, a suitable tube can be placed at the time of operation.

2. *Is the gastrointestinal tract functional?*
Intestinal obstruction or severe ileus contra-indicates the use of the enteral route. Similarly, if a suitable length of bowel does not exist, as in some cases of the short bowel syndrome, the parenteral route would be indicated. It cannot usually be predicted in malabsorption syndromes whether the gut will retain sufficient of its digestive and absorptive functions to enable the enteral route to be used. Those with diseases affecting the upper small intestine are likely to respond less well than a typical case of Crohn's disease where the terminal ileum alone is affected. In pancreatic and biliary disease the composition of the diet itself may largely determine whether it is effectively absorbed.

3. *Will the maximum tolerated gastrointestinal intake be sufficient?*
In catabolic states, as previously indicated, the intravenous route may have to be used simply because it is possible to administer greater amounts of nitrogen and energy in this way. Some studies in children with Crohn's disease have reported reversal of growth retardation after intravenous nutrition, but subsequent work has shown that the same results can be achieved by the enteral route.

4. *Is it the intention to provide complete bowel rest?*
The concept that resting the intestine from its mechanical digestive and absorptive functions by withholding all oral and enteral intake might enable a diseased bowel to heal has been studied in many patients with Crohn's disease. Nutrition is maintained by the parenteral route. None of the trials have been well controlled and it is not clear whether the bowel rest itself or the improvement in nutritional status is responsible for any benefit obtained from this type of treatment. There is greater rationale for resting the bowel in the case of fistulae. In Crohn's disease the consensus is that primary Crohn's fistulae do not respond well to this therapy and require surgical correction, but that there is a satisfactory response in postoperative fistulae.

Low residue enteral diets also provide effective bowel rest, certainly of the distal small intestine, and this is a more satisfactory approach than using parenteral nutrition because nutrients within the bowel lumen are important for the health of the mucosa. Low residue enteral diets are of value in the management of intestinal fistulae and often allow spontaneous closure to occur.

Parenteral nutrition may be used as an adjunct to standard medical treatment for severe ulcerative colitis, but never instead of it. It may prevent nutritional depletion resulting from the intense catabolic drive, and bowel rest may reduce the diarrhoea but does not induce remission of the disease.

Thus individual circumstances will largely determine whether one or more routes are used simultaneously. For example, when bowel rest or low residue is not important, the patient should be encouraged to eat normal meals in addition to enteral administration. Similarly, where the intravenous route is chosen to meet the heavy demands of catabolic states, oral nutrition may continue. If intravenous nutrition alone, for whatever reason, has been employed for more than a few days, simultaneous administration of an enteral diet will allow recovery of mucosal function before a normal diet is resumed.

5. *How long should nutritional support be maintained?*
Before embarking on nutritional treatment it is wise to define the end-point of the course. If restitution of a nutritional deficit is the sole aim, attainment of nutritional parameters within 10% of ideal is reasonable. In other circumstances a more arbitrary end-point would be necessary; it might be decided that 2 weeks' pre-operative nutritional therapy is a reasonable compromise between the need for surgery and the restoration of nutrition. In conditions such as neurological dysphagia the end-point can be defined as recovery of function. This will apply also to extensive disease or resection of the small intestine. What cannot be predicted is when recovery will occur, if ever. In cases like this, permanent nutritional support may be necessary.

Nutritional Support at Home

In cases where permanent nutritional support is required, consideration of numerous factors will be necessary. Administration of parenteral nutrition in the home is complex. Enteral feeding at home is relatively easy, and improvisation can produce satisfactory results. Parenteral nutrition has been successfully used in the home on numerous occasions and for many years but requires careful supervision from an appropriate centre. In some units, where local circumstances create a high demand, special programmes for patients' education have been instituted. Despite the potential for serious complications, many of the home parenteral nutritional programmes have been highly successful. However, the decision to implement such a course should not be taken lightly.

Oral Feeding

There are four types of complete nutritional preparations for oral feeding, namely blenderised food, hospital-prepared liquid diets, proprietary whole protein preparations and elemental diets.

Blenderised Diets

Simply blenderising the normal diet may be all that is required if there is some restriction of swallowing. The large volume of fluid required to blenderise whole food may be unacceptable to some patients.

Hospital-Prepared Liquid Diets and Proprietary Whole Protein Preparations

The choice between hospital-prepared liquid diets and proprietary whole protein preparations (Table 13.1) is by no means clear-cut. In favour of the former is that they are cheaper and can be made to suit the individual patient's requirements. However, hospital-prepared diets are usually milk based and although the composition of their major constituents is usually known, a full vitamin or trace element profile may not be available. This lack of information assumes importance when the diets are the sole nutritional intake and when they are used in patients with conditions which are likely to produce vitamin and/or trace metal deficiencies.

Not all hospitals are equipped with a diet kitchen and if the cost of this facility is added to the cost of the constituents of the diet, the commercial preparations are economically competitive. Immediate availability of the ready-made whole

Table 13.1. Some proprietary whole protein feeds

Product	Non-protein kilocalorie:nitrogen (g)	Osmolality	Lactose content (g/litre)	Comments
Clinifeed ISO (Roussel)	200:1	270[a]	18.7	Standard Roussel tube feed. 375 ml per can Clinifeed 400, Favour, Protein rich and Select also available
Ensure (Abbott)	154:1	450	Nil	Diarrhoea, possibly less of a problem than with others Small containers (235 ml). Very palatable. May need calorie supplementation Ensure Plus, high nitrogen feed, also available
Isocal (Mead Johnson)	170:1	350	Nil	Very similar to Ensure 355 ml per can
Nutrauxil (Kabi Vitrum)	140:1	350	0.1	Available in bottles of 200 ml for sip feeding and 500 ml for direct connection to delivery system
Triosorbon (BDH)	130:1	250[a,b]	1.5[b]	Rich in medium chain triglycerides Low energy content. Comes as powder

[a] Osmolarity
[b] Made up to give 1 kcal (total) per ml

protein diet is a considerable advantage and saves much nursing time in administration. In the few patients who may be lactose intolerant a non-milk based commercial diet should be used.

Elemental Diets

The indications for elemental diets will be discussed below, but oral administration poses problems of patient compliance due to their unpalatability. The unpleasant proteinaceous smell is due to organic amino acids and only limited success has been achieved in disguising the taste by commercial flavourings.

Flavourings are made available by the manufacturers of commercial elemental diets but it should be noted that these increase osmolarity and alter the pH of the solutions. Some workers have experimented with their own flavourings, adding fruit juices, teas, soups and spices, but the use of some of these detracts from the elemental nature of the diets.

A total prescribed daily intake should be divided into eight feeds and given to the patients individually at 2-hourly intervals.

Enteral Nutrition

The use of a fine-bore catheter for gastrointestinal feeding is not a new concept. Fallis and Barron reported their experience with polyethylene tubes with an outside diameter of 1.9 mm in 1952 and found that they were well tolerated for several months. More recently, the development of silicone elastomer catheters has increased the comfort for prolonged feeding.

Surgically Placed Catheters

If postoperative enteral nutrition is indicated, an appropriate catheter can be sited at the time of operation through an oesophagostomy, gastrostomy or jejunostomy, depending on the circumstances.

Nasally Passed Catheters

Although large-bore tubes are easier to pass than fine tubes, the latter are more comfortable and any initial reluctance on the part of the patient to undergo the procedure is rapidly forgotten and tolerance for long periods is customary. The flexibility of modern catheters sometimes allows them to coil in the oesophagus when being passed. This can be avoided by prefreezing the tube or by using a stilette. Several catheters now have a mercury olive at the distal end, which allows greater ease of placement.

The tube should be marked at approximately 55 cm and passage to this mark will enable it to reach well into the body of the stomach. That the catheter has passed safely into the stomach can be confirmed at the bedside by injecting 30 ml air through the tube and auscultating over the epigastrium. It is wise to use a radio-opaque catheter so that its position can be checked by X-ray before infusion of the diet. If nasojejunal placement is required, a further length of the feeding tube is passed into the stomach and an appropriate interval allowed for the catheter to negotiate the pylorus and travel to the jejunum. A plain radiograph of the abdomen for confirmation of correct positioning should be obtained before commencement of the infusion. Alternatively, the whole procedure can be performed using intermittent radiographic screening if the facilities are available. Recently direct endoscopic placement of the catheter in the duodenum has been advocated.

Both intragastric and intrajejunal administration of elemental diet have been widely used with good results but each route has disadvantages. A nasogastric tube is quicker and easier to pass but the hypertonicity of the solution may lead to gastric retention. It has been suggested that the stomach should be aspirated twice daily and the infusion discontinued for a few hours if the gastric aspirate exceeds 300 ml. On the other hand, because of side-effects related to hyperosmolarity, initial jejunal infusion should be more dilute.

Selection of Enteral Diet

There are many proprietary preparations available for enteral feeding, most ready for immediate administration (Table 13.1).

Whole Protein Preparations

These are cheaper and should be used in preference to elemental diets, which should be reserved for specific indications. Although many of the preparations are almost identical, there are a number of features which should be critically assessed.

The diet should provide all the essential nutrients in quantities at least sufficient to meet the Recommended Dietary Allowances. This is particularly important with respect to trace metals and vitamins, which should be present in generous amounts as many of the patients in whom the diets will be used may have specific deficiencies.

The osmolarity of the full strength preparations should ideally be less than 400 mosmol/litre to obviate the need for prolonged starter regimes. In general, diarrhoea due to the high osmolarity of the feed is less of a problem than previously thought, though it can occasionally be troublesome.

A suitable ratio of nitrogen to non-protein energy content should be chosen for the patient. Normal, well-nourished, well-compensated man makes efficient use of nitrogen and requires approximately 350 non-protein kilocalories (1.46 MJ) for every gram of nitrogen. Recent work in patients receiving intravenous nutrition has suggested that a severely catabolic patient, although requiring more total calories, requires proportionately much more nitrogen in the ratio of non-protein kilocalories to nitrogen of 130:1 (0.54 MJ:1). For most hospitalised non-catabolic patients a ratio of between 200 (0.84 MJ:1) and 250:1 (1.05 MJ:1) is best. Many of the proprietary preparations have energy to nitrogen ratios of below 200, but it is a simple procedure to add a glucose polymer solution to increase calorie content.

Finally, there has to be consideration of whether a lactose-free diet is required. Although it is true that many adults, particularly of Asian or African origin, have low lactose levels in their intestinal brush borders, the problem of lactose intolerance has been overestimated in the past. Many acute intestinal illnesses are complicated by a temporary lactose intolerance and in these patients it is wiser to select a non-milk based preparation.

Elemental Diets

The elemental diets became available for widespread use before the developments in enteral administration and subsequent expansion of the range of proprietary whole protein based diets. Consequently elemental diets have been advocated in many circumstances where the cheaper whole protein preparation would suffice. Low residue is a feature of both types of nutritional support and many of the benefits previously claimed for elemental diets can be attributed to this characteristic. It has been claimed that elemental diets are more easily absorbed than polymeric food because hydrolysis is not required. Theoretically this might be advantageous in special cases such as exocrine pancreatic insufficiency or the short bowel syndrome but there are no well controlled data to support this assertion. Recent work has demonstrated that small peptides are absorbed from the intestinal lumen, often with a kinetic advantage over free amino acids.

A number of uncontrolled studies have suggested that elemental diets are effective in inducing a remission in Crohn's disease. Because the patients involved have usually been subjected to bed rest as well as standard medical treatment, it is not possible to attribute improvement directly to the elemental diet. At the moment there seems to be no strong indication for the use of elemental diets as a method of inducing remission of the active disease process.

Administration

The sudden administration of a large volume of concentrated feed of high osmolality to a patient whose previous gastrointestinal intake was minimal is likely to provoke intolerance with vomiting, abdominal cramps and diarrhoea. For this reason it is customary to use a "starter diet" with gradual increase in volume and concentration. A suggested regime using the proprietary preparation, Ensure, is shown in Table 13.2.

It may take longer to reach full strength using elemental diets because of their osmolality. If the patient shows signs of intolerance, reduction to the

Table 13.2. Starter diet progressing to full strength using Ensure and glucose polymer Caloreen[a]

Day	ml	Ensure Cans	Caloreen	N_2 (g)	Non-protein energy (kilocalories)	Total volume ml	Comments
1	705	3	60 g	4.2	870	1500	Half strength. Water added to provide total volume
2	1175	5	100 g	6.95	1450	2000	Two-thirds strength
3	1645	7	350 ml 40% solution	9.8	2040	1995	Full strength

Continue as per day 3 unless additional nitrogen and energy required, when regimes for days 4 and 5 are invoked

Day	ml	Ensure Cans	Caloreen	N_2 (g)	Non-protein energy (kilocalories)	Total volume ml	Comments
4	2115	9	450 ml 40% solution	12.6	2620	2565	—
5	2585	11	550 ml 40% solution	15.4	3205	3135	—

[a] Added in proportions shown, Caloreen adjusts non-protein kilocalorie to nitrogen ratio to 200:1

previous day's volume and concentration should be undertaken until the patient can tolerate the higher dose.

Although it is possible to infuse a feed over the entire 24 h, for ambulatory patients it is reasonable to allow a break during waking hours. Although infusion of the diet does not interfere with sleep in most patients, it is safer to avoid nocturnal feeding in the elderly. Enteral intake should be adjusted to give a positive balance of about 5 g nitrogen.

Infusion of the diet can be controlled by a gravity drip method or by a pump. The former is simple but less reliable, especially when supervision is poor. The use of a pump is more usual and permits administration of the diet during sleep. A number of inexpensive commercially manufactured pumps specifically designed for enteral nutrition administration is available.

The control afforded by a reliable pump allows continuous infusion of the diet over 18–24 h daily and this is undoubtedly the technique of choice. It results in better patient tolerance of the diet and is more efficient in the use of nursing time than repeated bolus administration, which has been shown to significantly delay gastric emptying, with the risk of nausea, vomiting and aspiration.

The use of a reservoir which can accommodate a complete day's nutrition reduces nursing time but some commercial preparations are supplied in a container that can be connected directly to the infusion set, and most are simple and easy to use. Theoretically there is a danger of infection if a large quantity of highly nutritious liquid is left for 24 h at room temperature. Although one or two reports of contamination and resultant infection exist, in practice this seems rare. A compromise might be to use a reservoir which can be filled with a limited quantity of feed, say, four times daily. In this way neither the infusion set nor the patient is disturbed. The time taken is small and the opportunity can be used to check that the whole system is working well.

Complications of Enteral Nutrition

It is important to be aware of the potential hazards of enteral nutrition so that early recognition will enable appropriate measures to be taken.

Tube-Related Complications

The use of flexible, fine-bore feeding tubes has effectively eliminated the problems of oesophageal ulceration, haemorrhage and stricture formation previously associated with the larger, more rigid Ryle's tubes. However, it is easy to pass a fine tube into the trachea, especially in an unconscious patient, or for the tube to coil up in the pharynx. Complications that would arise from infusion of feed in such cases can be avoided by always checking that the tube is in the stomach.

Aspiration

Gastro-oesophageal reflux was frequently a problem of large-calibre tubes, but fine-bore tubes do not interfere with the anti-reflux mechanisms. The incidence of aspiration is of the order of 3%, but only one fatality attributable to this complication has been reported. Elderly, obtunded and unconscious patients are most at risk, particularly when there is a pulmonary problem. The hazard can be minimised by slow pump-controlled, continuous feeding to prevent accumulation in the stomach, by raising the head of the bed or sitting the patient at an angle of 30°, or by administering the diet into the jejunum.

Gastrointestinal Side-effects

Nausea, vomiting, abdominal cramps and distension are usually minor problems that can be alleviated by a reduction in the rate of infusion. Gastric retention is not usually troublesome during administration rates of less than 125 ml per hour, and the problem can be avoided by bypassing the stomach with intrajejunal feeding.

Diarrhoea is rarely troublesome, even with the high osmolalities of the elemental diet. When it does occur, other causes such as concurrent antibiotic therapy should be excluded. The use of milk-based formulations in lactose-deficient patients and the bacterial contamination of the enteric feed are other possibilities.

Metabolic Complications

The high-carbohydrate content of many of the enteric preparations introduces a danger of osmotic diuresis secondary to hyperglycaemia and glycosuria. In catabolic patients there is a relative insulin lack and it may be necessary to give insulin to such patients during feeding. Diabetics, even those previously controlled on oral hypoglycaemic agents, may need insulin during a period of enteral feeding and this is best administered by a continuous infusion. Failure to maintain normoglycaemia may surprise the unaware by the rapid development of hyperosmolar coma. A high protein intake may also lead to hyperosmolar dehydration; the nitrogen arising from 100 g of protein requires 1.7 litres of water to be excreted as isotonic urea and unrestricted access to water is mandatory if this complication is to be avoided.

Electrolyte Disturbances

Electrolyte disturbances are more likely to be related to the underlying disorder but the anabolic response stimulated by the feeding may exacerbate the abnormalities by shifting ions from the extracellular to intracellular compartments.

Nutritional Problems

Most proprietary enteric preparations are nutritionally satisfactory but compliance with the recommended dietary intake is not sufficient in all patients. Anabolic patients will have increased requirements for potassium and zinc, and many patients in whom enteral feeding is indicated have certain deficiencies, particularly of vitamins and trace elements, secondary to the underlying disease process. Some elemental diets have very little fat and may lead to essential fatty acid deficiency.

Liver Function Abnormalities

Occasionally abnormalities in liver function tests occur; these include elevations of hepatocellular enzymes, alkaline phosphatase and bilirubin.

Parenteral Nutrition

The institution of parenteral nutrition is a major procedure which should not be undertaken lightly. Neither must it be withheld when there are sound indications. The basis of all indications for parenteral nutrition, with the controversial exception of the provision of bowel rest, is the inability to provide satisfactory support via the gastrointestinal tract. The large number of products available for parenteral nutrition, the poor understanding of simple nutritional principles and the variety and serious nature of potential complications make what is essentially a simple procedure unnecessarily complicated for many physicians.

Selection of Solution

In a similar way to enteral feeding, nutritional requirements consist of an adequate balance of nitrogen and energy, supplemented by trace elements, vitamins and electrolytes.

Nitrogen Source

The previously available protein hydrolysates have largely been replaced by synthetic L-amino acid solutions. These are available with or without electrolytes and certain products have particular advantages. Synthamin (Travenol Laboratories) contains some phosphate, an essential component of an intravenous feeding regime which is often omitted. Vamin (Kabivitrum) is available with or without glucose. The major differences, however, lie in the amino acid composition of the different solutions. Synthamin, which is cheaper and has the advantage of being available in concentrations of 7, 9, 14 and 17 g nitrogen per litre, has a relatively high content of the inexpensive amino acids alanine and glycine but a lower proportion of essential amino acids than Vamin, which is based on egg protein, or Aminoplex 12 (Geistlich), which is modelled on Rose's recommendations for amino acid requirements. Whether these differences are clinically important has not been established. In practice it is better for a clinician to work with one or perhaps two preparations and to become familiar with their composition.

Energy Source

Carbohydrates, Polyols and Ethanol

Glucose is the simplest carbohydrate source of energy and can be utilised by every cell in the body. A number of alternatives are available, including other carbohydrates, polyols such as sorbitol, xylitol and glycerol which can be converted to true carbohydrates, and ethanol. Although the use of highly concentrated glucose solutions may have side-effects, in general such solutions are superior to these substances, to which only a brief reference will be made here.

Fructose: Fructose does not stimulate an insulin response and inhibits gluconeogenesis in the liver, so sparing amino acids. However, it cannot be utilised as such by the brain but requires transformation to glucose. About 70% of the fructose undergoes this transformation and insulin is, therefore, required for its further metabolism. Rapid metabolism of fructose may cause lactic acidosis and hyperuricaemia.

Sorbitol: Sorbitol has no advantages over fructose, to which it is converted by the enzyme sorbitol dehydrogenase.

Ethanol: Ethanol has a high calorific value, supplying 7 Cal per gram (0.029 MJ/g), but the body can utilise only 2.4 g/kg per day. Like fructose and sorbitol, it carries a risk of precipitating lactic acidosis and because of its well-known pharmacological and toxic effects is best avoided.

Glucose: Glucose has several advantages over the above. All tissues can metabolise glucose; indeed, it is the only carbohydrate which can be utilised by the brain. Glucose stimulates insulin secretion and promotes an anabolic response. Problems may arise in postoperative and catabolic states, in which insulin resistance may develop, and to prevent hyperglycaemia exogenous insulin must be added. Failure to do so may result in the hyperosmolar syndrome with excessive glucose-induced osmotic diuresis and dehydration. The requirements at the bedside for insulin vary, and repeated monitoring of plasma glucose may be necessary with adjustment of insulin dosage. The high endogenous insulin levels produced during infusion of 50% glucose solutions may on its cessation cause reactive hypoglycaemia; this can be avoided by the infusion of a 5% glucose solution. Awareness of these potential hazards allows high concentrations to be given with safety in the majority of patients. For intravenous nutrition it is the carbohydrate of choice.

Fat

The advantage of fat as an energy source is its high calorific value, approximately 9 Cal/g (0.038 MJ/g), so that a large amount of energy can be given in a small volume. It is isotonic and can be given by a peripheral vein. The direct infusion of the fat into the venous system mimics closely the way fat is normally obtained from the gut, when, having been absorbed, it passes via the lymphatic system and the thoracic duct into the left subclavian vein. Modern fat emulsions based on soya bean oil are certainly free from the side-effects of the earlier cottonseed oil preparations, which led to their being banned in the United States. Most of the recent studies have been performed using Intralipid (Kabivitrum) and only this solution will be referred to. The ability to clear Intralipid from the circulation varies depending on the patient's condition. Severely ill patients, especially those with septicaemia, may have low clearance rates, and accumulation in the liver and reticuloendothelial system generally may also be more of a problem in these patients. Heparin has been shown to promote clearance.

Work on the utilisation of fat as an energy source is difficult to interpret. It is known that there is an essential amount of carbohydrate required for nitrogen sparing to occur but above this level fat can be a useful source of calories. However, if fat is to be used as a major calorie source, a period of adaptation is necessary before it can be utilised to advantage.

Failure to provide any fat will result in essential fatty acid deficiency which may cause skin rashes after several weeks. Fat is also a vehicle for the administration of fat-soluble vitamins. A previously suggested advantage that the phospholipid content protects against hypophosphataemia is no longer tenable.

Intralipid is expensive and cannot reliably be mixed with other nutrients. It is, however, an acceptable alternative energy source in non-septic patients. A fat-free period of at least 6 h should be maintained each day and blood checked for lipaemia after this period by inspecting a centrifuged specimen for opalescence. Blood for biochemical monitoring should be taken at this time as lipaemia interferes with many analyses.

Vitamins and Minerals

The daily requirements are not known with certainty, especially in the artificial circumstances of parenteral nutrition and in the widely different clinical situations. A combination of the use of proprietary preparations of vitamin and mineral supplements, regular biochemical monitoring and strong clinical awareness of the potential for deficiencies will prevent any serious problems.

Folic acid is required for metabolism involving the transference of one-carbon units such as the synthesis of purines and pyrimidines, which is promoted by amino acid infusions, especially methionine, and an anabolic response generally. The body's stores of folic acid are poor and failure to provide this vitamin will result in thrombocytopenic anaemia and leucopenia within 1–2 weeks of starting intravenous nutrition.

Zinc deficiency has received much attention in the literature due to its occurrence during long periods of parenteral nutrition in which trace elements were not supplied. Florid deficiency results in skin rashes and hair loss, but as zinc is involved in the metabolism of over 70 enzymes, subclinical deficiency is just as important. Although plasma and urinary zinc measurements are not a good guide to zinc status, very low levels do indicate true deficiency. This can be avoided by the administration of at least 50 μmol/day, which is more than that contained in most proprietary preparations.

Hypophosphataemia during intravenous nutrition has been widely documented and although absolute requirements are not laid down the supply should be guided by regular monitoring.

Administration

Administration of concentrated glucose solutions requires access to a large fast-flowing central vein. One of the most suitable for parenteral nutrition is a subclavian vein reached by the infraclavicular route. Many types of catheters are available, but those made out of silicone elastomer are superior because of their less irritant effect on the vessel wall and because their lightness and extreme flexibility enables them to "float" in the centre of the bloodstream. These features allow a longer life with fewer complications. The catheter is passed into the vein through a plastic cannula which is itself inserted into the vessel over a needle of slightly longer length. Some types require the plastic cannula to be left in situ although it should be withdrawn from the vein. Some catheters have removable hubs which facilitate complete removal of the plastic cannula and also construction of a skin tunnel if this is necessary.

The catheter tip should lie in the superior vena cava just above the right atrium. This can be estimated or the whole procedure performed under radiographic screening, which is useful in manipulation of a catheter intent on passing up the internal jugular vein. In either case a penetrated chest X-ray should be performed on completion to confirm the catheter tip position and to exclude pneumothorax, which is a well-recognised but, in experienced hands, rare complication.

The construction of a skin tunnel prolongs catheter life and reduces the risk of infection. It often enables a catheter to be fixed more securely and dressing is made easier.

There is a difference of opinion over the frequency with which the catheter entry site should be dressed, ranging from daily care to the use of transparent dressings which allow inspection and are changed when necessary. Once to twice weekly is probably acceptable with full aseptic precautions and a swab taken if inflammation is present. It is not necessary to change a catheter which is working well in an apyrexial patient. If infection does arise, early removal with the insertion of a new catheter on the opposite side is required.

One of the aims of parenteral nutrition is to simulate normal nutrient provision and it is therefore beneficial to infuse the energy source concurrently with the nitrogen source. This is achieved by the use of a "V" shaped infusion set manufactured as one unit allowing mixture just before joining the catheter. The use of this is to be recommended over adaptors or three-way taps, where the extra connection involved increases the risk of infection. Three-in-one, so-called "W" infusion sets are also available. It should be emphasised that the feeding catheter and the infusion set should not be used for other purposes, such as injection of drugs, blood transfusion, central venous pressure measurements or the taking of blood. Although it is possible to provide parenteral nutrition without any other elaborate apparatus using a simple gravity drip method and the individual bottles of nutrient solutions, two technological developments are worth consideration:

1. *Pumps*. In adult medicine extreme accuracy of volume and timing is rarely necessary, but control of the infusions is made safer and simpler by the use of pumps. Inadvertent rapid infusion of concentrated glucose solutions is more likely to occur on a general ward at night, when nursing supervision may be reduced, leading rapidly to dehydration and hyperosmolar coma. This is prevented by using intravenous pumps which are equipped with alarm systems; these are, however, expensive. Air embolus is prevented and the infusion is kept to time. The slight positive pressure helps to keep the fine-bore catheter patent and spontaneous blockage is thereby prevented. Most models incorporate a rechargeable battery, allowing ambulant patients freedom of movement. Pumps are particularly helpful when used in conjunction with the once daily large bag system.

2. *Once daily bag system*. The unsatisfactory necessity of changing the nutrient solutions every 8 h or so, along with the addition on the ward of insulin, trace elements and vitamin mixtures to the solutions, has led to a system which avoids these potentially dangerous procedures. A sterile 3-litre bag is made up in the pharmacy under laminar flow conditions, containing all the glucose and amino acid solutions and all the additives prescribed for a 24-h period. Some centres now add Intralipid to this, but there is concern about interfering with the droplet size of the fat emulsion and most clinicians prefer to administer the fat separately. The bag is sealed after one limb of the infusion set has been inserted and the whole unit is transported to the ward, where it is set up at a time to coincide with the dressing of the catheter site. This greatly

reduces the potential for infection and is less demanding of nursing time. Ideally the patient undergoing parenteral nutrition only requires one intervention every 24 h.

Designing a Regime

The detailed prescription of a parenteral nutrition regime depends on the circumstances of the patient. Renal failure, severe trauma, sepsis or gross electrolyte upset may require daily adjustments of intake depending upon the result of biochemical monitoring. Less severely ill and more stable patients will be able to cope with the same regime repeated every 24 h. There are, however, a number of guiding principles when designing such a regime.

For non-catabolic patients, particularly those who are severely mal-nourished but who have adjusted to their starved state metabolically, 0.2 g nitrogen per kilogram of actual body weight is a reasonable nitrogen intake with which to commence feeding. Nitrogen supplies can be adjusted according to simple nitrogen balance estimations (see under "Monitoring" below) to give a positive balance of at least 5 g. Catabolic patients are liable to need much greater amounts, for example a 50-kg man who has sustained 40% burns may require up to 30 g nitrogen per day.

The total non-nitrogen calories supplied also depends upon the catabolic state of the patient. The principles of energy supply discussed under "Selection of Enteral Diet" apply to intravenous requirements.

Where fat is chosen as the main energy source approximately 30% of non-protein calories should be given as carbohydrate, and a maximum of 5 g of Intralipid per kilogram is recommended. In practice a check should be made that the patient is able to clear the fat from the plasma within 8 h and in septic patients only that amount necessary to satisfy essential fatty acid requirements should be used.

The provision of 5 mmol potassium and 1 mmol magnesium for each gram of nitrogen is a reasonable starting intake for these intracellular cations, later adjustments being dependent on biochemical parameters.

Parenteral nutrition regimes run smoothly if prescriptions are written on a 24-h basis. Whilst intensive care units are equipped to deal with daily modifications of prescription, on a general ward it is useful to have a master chart on which the day-by-day prescription is entered (Fig. 13.1).

Complications of Parenteral Nutrition

The list of potential complications of intravenous nutrition is daunting and emphasises the need for rigorous attention to detail in both institution of the feeding and monitoring of progress.

Complications of Catheter Insertion

In experienced hands complications are rare. Routine use of the head-down position in association with the Valsalva manoeuvre will prevent air embolism.

PARENTERAL NUTRITION

NAME _John Smith_   DATE _24 · 1 · 83_

LINE A				LINE B			
Time	Solution and additives	Vol.	Rate.	Time	Solution and additives	Vol.	Rate
0600	Synthamin 14 with electrolytes + 1 ampoule Solivito	500ml	8 hrly	0600	50% dextrose + insulin as directed	500ml	8 hrly
1400	Synthamin 14 with electrolytes + 1 ampoule addamel	500ml	8 hrly	1400	50% dextrose + insulin as directed	500ml	8 hrly
2200	Travenol solution A	500ml	8 hrly	2200	10% Intralipid + 1 ampoule vitlipid	500ml	8 hrly

Further Instructions

1. See separate instructions for insulin infusion
2. Change infusion set daily and dressing twice weekly at 1400 hrs.

Fig. 13.1. Master chart for parenteral nutrition.

Infusion into the pleural space should never occur if confirmation is obtained that the catheter is in the vascular system by lowering the bag below the bed and watching for retrograde flow. A rare complication is superior vena cava thrombosis. This is usually the result of long-standing feeding and presumably due to a combination of the presence of a foreign body (the catheter) in the vein and the infusion of concentrated glucose solutions.

Sepsis

Sepsis is by far the most frequent and potentially serious complication. All the precautions of catheter insertion, preparation of the infusion solutions and care of the site are designed to prevent it. A carefully kept temperature chart is mandatory so that early action can be taken if a pyrexia develops. Other sources of infection should be excluded by clinical examination, blood, sputum and urine cultures and appropriate X-rays. A swab should be taken from the catheter entry site and if no other source of infection becomes apparent within 24 h, the catheter should be removed. If positive blood cultures are obtained and the pyrexia continues after removing the catheter, appropriate antibiotics should be instituted. Culture of the catheter tip for both bacteria and fungi may help in antibiotic selection.

Metabolic Complications

The most important metabolic complication is hyperglycaemia, with glycosuria and osmotic diuresis. This may progress to hyperosmolar non-ketotic coma if careful monitoring is neglected. Known diabetics (and latent diabetics) and patients in severe catabolic states with relative insulin lack are most at risk and require careful control of exogenous insulin infusion. Reactive hypoglycaemia may occur if concentrated glucose infusions are not followed by a dilute dextrose solution. Fructose, sorbitol and ethanol may be complicated by lactic acidosis and hyperchloraemic acidosis is a frequent complication of infusion of large quantities of amino acid hydrochlorides. When parenteral nutrition is the sole source of nutrition for prolonged periods, deficiency states may develop. Hypophosphataemia causes an increased affinity of oxygen for haemoglobin, impairing transport of oxygen to tissues. Trace element deficiency, particularly zinc deficiency, may occur in an anabolic phase if not adequately supplied.

Liver Problems

Jaundice is a frequent but transient problem of unknown cause. Cholestatic syndromes have been widely reported and may be due to lack of stimulation of the gall bladder in patients whose gut is not being used. Rises in transaminases are also frequent and one report has attributed the development of cirrhosis to parenteral nutrition.

Monitoring

There are three aspects of patient monitoring during nutritional support. The early detection of metabolic and other complications is of greater importance in the parenterally fed patients but should not be neglected in enteral nutrition. Deficiency states may arise when the period of feeding is prolonged and normal oral intake withheld. Finally, documenting nutritional response is important to allow appropriate changes in the regime.

Once weekly blood and urine collection is adequate for a patient on enteral feeding but it is recommended that estimation of plasma glucose urea and electrolytes and liver function tests be carried out twice weekly for parenteral nutrition. All patients starting nutritional support should have their glucose status carefully monitored. Six-hourly urinalysis for the first 24 h and once daily thereafter is adequate for enteral nutrition, but on commencing parenteral nutrition a plasma glucose profile followed by 6-hourly urine testing is recommended. The longer and more dependent the patient is on either enteral or parenteral nutritional support the greater should be the awareness both clinically and biochemically of deficiency states. Once weekly full blood count, serum iron, B_{12} and folic acid should be measured. Calcium, phosphate, magnesium and the trace elements copper and zinc (and other trace elements if available) should also be estimated in blood. Vitamin assays are helpful if available, but clinical awareness and an adequate supply should prevent complications. Measurements of urinary electrolytes and trace elements can assist in assessing deficiency states. Initial nutritional assessment has been referred to above. Once weekly anthropometric and serum protein measurements are useful, and a repetition of skin tests on completion of the course may show conversion from anergy to immunocompetence due to nutritional improvement. Assessment of weekly nitrogen balance is important for determining the adequacy of the nutritional regime. If a positive balance of several grams is not found, there is a need for an increase in nitrogen supply. Although it is possible to measure total urine and faecal nitrogen, the methods are cumbersome and great accuracy is not required for nutritional monitoring. A simple measurement of urinary urea excretion can be used based on the following assumptions:

1. Faecal nitrogen excretion is fairly constant at 1–2 g daily in the absence of diarrhoea, even in severe catabolic illnesses.

2. The majority of nitrogen in urine is present as urea. Based on these assumptions the formula

$$\text{nitrogen excretion (g)} = \frac{\text{urine urea (mmol)}}{30} + 2$$

can be satisfactorily used. Nitrogen intake can be calculated from the nitrogen content of the parenteral or enteral nutrient solutions. If patients are also taking a normal diet careful recording of the intake over the 24-h period during which the urine is collected will enable the nitrogen content to be calculated.

Nutritional Aspects of Liver Disease

Patients with chronic liver disease are frequently malnourished, although the presence of oedema and ascites may mask this if body weight alone is used to assess nutritional status. They are frequently anergic to immunological skin testing but factors other than nutritional are involved and it is not clear yet whether correction of nutritional deficit alone would restore immunocompetence. Visceral protein levels are reduced in patients with chronic liver disease, although, for example, albumin synthesis rates are frequently well preserved and depressed serum levels may be a reflection of malnutrition. For this reason patients with chronic liver disease without encephalopathy should be on a high protein diet. If nutritional support is indicated there is no contra-indication to using standard products and surprisingly large amounts of nitrogen are often well tolerated. Many patients with hepatic decompensation are erroneously treated with a low protein diet in the absence of encephalopathy.

Protein restriction is, of course, standard treatment in patients with hepatic encephalopathy. There is considerable controversy over the cause of hepatic encephalopathy and the role of certain nutritional products in its treatment. Recent attention has been drawn to the excess aromatic amino acids (AAAs) and reduced branched chain amino acids (BCAAs) in encephalopathic patients (and also cirrhotic patients without encephalopathy). The controversy centres around whether the administration of a solution rich in BCAAs is curative in encephalopathy by returning the AAA:BCAA ratio to normal. However, from the nutritional aspect BCAA-rich solutions may be better tolerated in encephalopathic patients and prevent the negative nitrogen balance ensuing from standard protein restriction treatment. Although these solutions have been administered intravenously in the work so far performed, the enteral route may be perfectly satisfactory. Enteral diets rich in BCAAs and low in AAAs are available but there is no data on their efficacy. Theoretically they may be of use in both chronic and acute hepatic encephalopathy. Finally there have been some reports that the ornithine salts of the branch chain keto acids may be beneficial.

Further Reading

Bistrian BR, Blackburn GL, Hallowell E, Heddle R (1974) Protein status of general surgical patients. JAMA 230: 858–860

Bistrian BR, Blackburn GL, Vitale J, Cochran D (1976) Prevalence of malnutrition in general medical patients. JAMA 235: 1567–1570

Blackburn GL, Kaminski MV (1980) Nutritional assessment and intravenous support. In: Karran SJ, Alberti KGMM (eds) Practical nutritional support. Pitman Medical, Tunbridge Wells, pp 166–189

Brown J (1981) Enteral feeds and delivery systems. Br J Hosp Med 26: 168–175

Driscoll RH, Rosenberg IH (1978) Total parenteral nutrition in inflammatory bowel disease. Med Clin North Am 62: 185–201

Fallis LS, Barron J (1952) Gastric and jejunal alimentation with fine polyethylene tubes. Arch Surg 65: 373

Hill GL, Blackett RL, Pickford I, Burkinshaw L, Young GA, Warren JV, Schorah CJ, Morgan DB (1978) Malnutrition in surgical patients—an unrecognised problem. Lancet I: 689

Jellife DB (1966) Assessment of the nutritional status of the community. WHO, Geneva

Johnston IDA, Lee HA (eds) (1979) Developments in clinical nutrition. MCS Consultants, Tunbridge Wells

Jung R (1981) Nutrition. Hosp Update 7: 883–898

Karran SJ, Alberti KGMM (eds) (1980) Practical nutritional support. Pitman Medical, Tunbridge Wells

Kirschner BS, Klich JR, Kalman SS, De Favaro MV, Rosenberg IH (1981) Reversal of growth retardation in Crohn's disease with therapy emphasising oral nutritional restitution. Gastroenterology 80: 10–15

Morin CL, Roulet M, Roy CC, Weber A (1980) Continuous elemental enteral alimentation in children with Crohn's disease and growth failure. Gastroenterology 79: 1205–1210

Powell-Tuck J (1978) Skin tunnel for central venous catheter: non-operative technique. Br Med J I: 625

Russel RI (ed) (1981) Elemental diets. CRC Press, Boca Raton

Shenkin A, Wretlind A (1978) Parenteral nutrition. World Rev Nutr Diet 28: 1

14 Drugs for Gastrointestinal Disease
C. J. C. Roberts and T. K. Daneshmend

Introduction

This section of the book is intended to provide the reader with concise information on the drugs used in the treatment of gastrointestinal disease. It will remind the prescribing physician about those factors which need to be considered when deciding to prescribe one of the drugs. Drug interactions and precautions are highlighted. A wider discussion about the indications and usefulness of the agent will be found in the earlier chapters of the book, to which the reader will be referred. In this chapter the drugs and drug groups are arranged in alphabetical order for ease of access.

Antacids

Antacids are used to relieve symptoms in oesophageal reflux (see Chap. 1) and in the treatment of peptic ulcer disease (see Chap. 2). Their therapeutic effect is brought about solely by chemical neutralisation of gastric acid. They differ in their neutralising capacity, their effect on bowel action, their sodium content and their cost. There are many proprietary mixtures, but the basic ingredients are sodium bicarbonate, aluminium hydroxide, magnesium hydroxide, magnesium trisilicate and calcium carbonate. In general the liquid preparations are more rapidly effective than tablets, but the latter have the advantage of convenience.

Neutralising Capacity

Sodium bicarbonate has a great capacity for neutralising gastric acid but its effect is short lived. Chemical reaction leads to free carbon dioxide, causing flatulence, and sodium chloride, which is absorbed. Sodium bicarbonate tends to cause systemic alkalosis. Of the longer-acting agents magnesium hydroxide is the most potent. It reacts with the hydrochloric acid rapidly to form the poorly absorbed magnesium chloride. When present in excessive amounts magnesium hydroxide can raise gastric pH to over 9.0.

Aluminium hydroxide also reacts rapidly with hydrochloric acid to form the poorly absorbed salt, aluminium chloride. When present in excess, gastric pH is only elevated to approximately 4.5. Aluminium hydroxide inhibits gastric smooth muscle contraction, delays gastric emptying, and is said to bind pepsin. There is also inhibition of intestinal smooth muscle contraction, which is thought to be due to interference with calcium fluxes by the trivalent aluminium ion. Aluminium hydroxide binds bile acids and phosphate within the gastrointestinal tract. The latter action has been used to reduce hypophosphataemia in patients with renal disease.

Calcium carbonate is a moderately potent antacid reacting in the stomach to form calcium chloride. It is capable of raising gastric pH to 7.5. Calcium within the gut stimulates the release of gastrin and this probably accounts for the acid rebound, a phenomenon sometimes seen in patients following calcium carbonate.

Magnesium trisilicate reacts only slowly with gastric hydrochloric acid to produce magnesium chloride and silicon dioxide. It is capable of raising the gastric pH to 6.0.

Pharmacokinetics

The only antacid to be freely absorbed is sodium bicarbonate. However, small amounts of the other cations are absorbed so that aluminium excretion may rise several-fold in normal individuals taking regular aluminium hydroxide. As much as 30% of the calcium in a dose of calcium carbonate may be absorbed and up to 10% of magnesium ions may be absorbed and subsequently renally excreted.

Adverse Effects

Aluminium ions tend to cause constipation, which has rarely led to intestinal obstruction. Nausea and vomiting have also been reported. Hypophosphataemia has occurred in patients on long-term aluminium hydroxide. Calcium carbonate has caused the milk–alkali syndrome, consisting of hypercalcaemia, renal calcinosis and chronic renal failure. Constipation and hypophosphataemia may also occur. The magnesium salts tend to cause diarrhoea and occasionally kidney stones have resulted from precipitation of absorbed silicates.

Special Considerations

Patients predisposed to oedematous states and hypertension should avoid preparations with a high sodium content. Patients with severe renal failure may not excrete the cations. An accumulation of aluminium may result in neurotoxicity, and hypermagnesaemia may lead to muscle weakness, hypotension and central nervous system depression. Antacids may interfere with the absorption of a number of concurrent drug therapies (see Chap. 1).

Prescribing Information

A large number of official and proprietary antacid preparations and mixtures are available. Aluminium hydroxide is available in tablets and mixture, both of which are very low in sodium. Magnesium hydroxide is available in mixture form containing very low amounts of sodium. Magnesium trisilicate is available as a mixture containing 6 mmol sodium/10 ml mixture. Magnesium trisilicate tablets, compound, contain both magnesium trisilicate and aluminium hydroxide and are low in sodium. The advantage of this tablet is that the effects of magnesium and aluminium on bowel habit tend to counteract one another. There is no official liquid preparation containing magnesium trisilicate and aluminium hydroxide without sodium. Proprietary preparations such as Gelusil suspension are available. Sodium bicarbonate is available as tablets. Calcium carbonate is not available in a single ingredient preparation but is found in many proprietary and official preparations. The reader is referred to the *British National Formulary* for a comprehensive list of recommended preparations.

Azathioprine

This drug is the preferred immunosuppressant for gastrointestinal disease. It has a place in the therapy of inflammatory bowel disease (see Chap. 5) and in chronic active hepatitis (see Chap. 8). Azathioprine is slowly converted to 6-mercaptopurine in the body. The action of the drug is firstly to block DNA and RNA synthetic pathways by feedback inhibition of phosphoribosylamine formation from glutamine and phosphoribosylpyrophosphate. In addition, lymphocyte rosette formation is suppressed with a predominant suppression of cell-mediated immune responses. Because of its immunosuppressant and antineoplastic actions, azathioprine is widely used in the treatment of malignancy and in the suppression of other harmful immune responses such as the graft reaction.

Pharmacokinetics

Azathioprine is completely absorbed from the gastrointestinal tract and is slowly converted into 6-mercaptopurine. 6-Mercaptopurine is eliminated from the body mainly after hepatic demethylation, desulphuration and also oxidation by xanthine oxidase. The elimination half-life of azathioprine is 3 h.

Adverse Effects

The most important adverse reaction to azathioprine is predictable bone marrow depression. Agranulocytosis, thrombocytopenia and aplastic anaemia are the inevitable consequences of excessive dosage. Providing the patient survives the acute attack the prognosis is usually good for bone marrow recovery. Other adverse effects include predisposition to malignancy with prolonged therapy and the occasional appearance of cholestatic jaundice. The drug is teratogenic and should not be used in patients who could become pregnant.

Special Considerations

Detoxification of 6-mercaptopurine is profoundly impaired in the presence of xanthine oxidase inhibitor such as allopurinol. Dose reduction to about one-third of the normal dose is mandatory in patients receiving this drug. Variability in dose requirements occurs in patients with hepatic disease because of impaired conversion of the drug. It is possible that this group is more susceptible to the hepatotoxic effects of the drug. Despite the widespread use of azathioprine in recent years it should not be forgotten that this drug is a highly toxic agent and the most careful clinical monitoring is required in patients taking the drug.

Prescribing Information

The dose of azathioprine which most clinicians employ is in the range of 1–3 mg/kg. It is advisable to start with a relatively low dose of the drug and to increase the dose whilst monitoring bone marrow function.

Bismuth Salts

Bismuth salts have been used in medicine for many years in dermatology, gastroenterology and the treatment of syphilis. In gastroenterology they have been used in the past as anti-diarrhoeal agents and have been found useful in patients with ileostomy to alter the consistency of the effluent. However, the only valid usage in modern gastroenterological practice is as second- or third-line therapy for peptic ulcer disease, where they are used in the commercially available preparation. De-Nol is a colloidal suspension of the bismuth salt which contains tripotassium dicitratobismuthate; it has been shown to have cytoprotective properties in that it partially prevents gastric ulcers in animals induced by ethanol, aspirin, phenylbutazone and stress. For a discussion of its indications, see Chap. 2. In man several well-controlled studies have suggested accelerated healing of both duodenal and gastric ulcers.

Pharmacokinetics

Orally administered bismuth remains virtually completely unabsorbed in the gastrointestinal tract and is excreted in the faeces. The minute amounts absorbed are excreted by the kidney.

Adverse Effects

The suspension tastes unpleasant and this may have an adverse effect on compliance. The tongue may be darkened. Bismuth has a constipating effect and causes darkening of the stools. This may be mistaken for melaena.

Special Considerations

Bismuth interferes with the absorption of tetracycline. It should not be administered to pregnant women and it is considered advisable to avoid bismuth in patients with severe renal failure for fear that accumulation of absorbed bismuth might have an adverse effect on the central nervous system.

Prescribing Information

De-Nol is a clear red liquid which contains 120 mg tripotassium dicitrato bismuthate in each 5 ml. A dose of 5 ml diluted with 15 ml water should be administered four times a day on a empty stomach 30 min before each of the three main meals and 2 h after the last meal of the day. The course should last for 28 days and a reassessment should be made. The dose may be increased and the course prolonged in resistant patients.

Carbenoxolone

Carbenoxolone is an ester of glycyrrhizinic acid derived from liquorice root. It has a steroid-like molecule. It has been found useful in the management of severe reflux oesophagitis, gastric ulcer and duodenal ulcer (see Chaps. 1, 2). Its most important clinical usage has been in the promoting of healing of gastric ulcers. Its mode of action is not entirely established but it has been shown to cause increases in the production and viscosity of gastric mucus and, in some studies, a reduction in the back diffusion of hyrogen ions across the gastric mucosa. The activities of pepsin, pepsinogen and chymotrypsin are reduced by the drug, but it has no effect on gastric acid output or gastric motility.

Pharmacokinetics

The drug is well absorbed, achieving peak levels in 1–2 h. Food interferes with carbenoxolone absorption so that the drug is best given before meals. The drug is 99% bound to plasma proteins. Elimination is by hepatic conjugation with glucuronic acid and excretion into bile. Plasma half-life is approximately 15 h in the healthy adult but may be prolonged in elderly patients.

Adverse Effects

The high incidence of adverse effects associated with this drug severely limits its usefulness. The most important of these are directly related to its mineralocorticoid action. Thus salt and water retention may exacerbate the fluid retention of cardiac failure and hepatic disease. Hypertensive control may be lost or frank hypertension precipitated by the drug. Profound hypokalaemia leading to muscle weakness, mental confusion and lethargy may also occur.

Special Considerations

Carbenoxolone should not be used in any patient liable to develop oedema. The elderly are particularly susceptible to the adverse effects and in general the drug should not be used in patients over the age of 65. It should be avoided if possible in the hypertensive patient and where hypokalaemia would be a dangerous occurrence, such as in the presence of digoxin therapy. Whilst spironolactone is capable of correcting the mineralocorticoid adverse effects of carbenoxolone, it has been shown to detract from the therapeutic effect and therefore should not be used. The use of thiazide diuretic, whilst alleviating the salt and water retention, will exacerbate the hypokalaemia. This hypokalaemia will not be amenable to treatment with slow-release potassium supplements. Concurrent amiloride or triamterene may be useful where carbenoxolone therapy is essential.

Prescribing Information

Carbenoxolone is available in three preparations.

   1. Carbenoxolone sodium 50 mg tablets for gastric ulcers (Biogastrone). The recommended dose is 100 mg three times daily after meals for 1 week, then 50 mg three times daily for 4–6 weeks.

   2. Positioned released carbenoxolone capsules 50 mg for duodenal ulceration (Duogastrone). The recommended dose is 50 mg four times a day, 20 min before meals for 6–12 weeks .

   3. For reflux oesophagitis, tablets containing carbenoxolone sodium 20 mg, alginic acid 600 mg, dried aluminium hydroxide 240 mg, magnesium trisilicate 60 mg, sodium bicarbonate 210 mg (Pyrogastrone). The adult dose is one tablet chewed three times daily immediately after meals and two at bedtime for 6 weeks. This expensive preparation probably has little advantage over antacids alone.

Chenodeoxycholic Acid

This primary dihydroxy bile acid is used in the medical treatment of cholesterol gall-stones. Indications for its use and mode of action are discussed in Chap. 7.

Pharmacokinetics

After oral administration it is rapidly absorbed, peak plasma levels being achieved within 80 min and blood levels being proportionate to dose. There is a 60% first pass clearance of chenodeoxycholic acid by the liver. Within the liver the drug is conjugated with glycine or taurine and is secreted into the bile and thence into the intestine. Within the intestine a small proportion is broken down by bacteria to lithocholic acid, which is mainly excreted by the kidney.

Adverse Effects

The most important adverse effect is diarrhoea, there being an incidence of 40%–50% in patients receiving a dose of 15 mg/kg body weight. Diarrhoea is caused by net water secretion within the colon, possibly secondary to colonic adenylcyclase activity. The onset of diarrhoea is usually within the first few weeks of therapy and may respond to a reduction in dosage. Hepatotoxicity has been a theoretical effect of chenodeoxycholic acid as both chenodeoxycholic acid and the bacterial breakdown product, lithocholic acid, have both been shown to be hepatotoxic in animal species. Although as many as 30% of patients may show a transient rise in serum transaminases (and in one study a two- to threefold rise was reported), fears of a serious hepatotoxicity in man seem unjustified.

Special Considerations

It has been suggested that chenodeoxycholic acid may have mild microsomal enzyme-inducing properties. Patients on oral anticoagulants, anti-epileptic therapy and oral hypoglycaemics should be monitored carefully when chenodeoxycholic acid therapy is started. Patients with inflammatory bowel disease and chronic liver disease, and pregnant women or those likely to become pregnant should not receive this therapy.

Prescribing Information

The dose of chenodeoxycholic acid is 10–15 mg/kg body weight daily, either as single or divided doses.

Cholestyramine

Cholestyramine is an ion exchange resin which is positively charged and which acts by binding substances within the gut lumen. It is used to reduce the pruritus associated with cholestatic jaundice by binding bile salts (see Chap. 8). It is also useful in the treatment of bile salt-induced diarrhoea. A further consequence of the drug's action is to increase the turnover rate of low-density lipoproteins and lower plasma cholesterol levels. This has been made use of in the treatment of familial hypercholesterolaemia.

Pharmacokinetics

Cholestyramine is hydrophilic but insoluble in water. In the gastrointestinal tract it remains unchanged, being unaffected by digestive enzymes and unabsorbed.

Adverse Effects

Nausea, vomiting, abdominal cramps and constipation are frequent occurrences. Hyperchloraemic acidosis due to absorption of the chloride ion has been reported in children. The binding of bile salts by cholestyramine may interfere with the absorption of fats, leading to steatorrhoea, and there may be impairment of absorption of fat-soluble vitamins. Osteomalacia and hypoprothombinaemia are uncommon side-effects of the drug consequent upon malabsorption of vitamins D and K respectively.

Special Considerations

Cholestyramine not only binds bile salts but may bind a number of acidic drugs and therefore prevent their absorption and effect. Most notable examples are oral anticoagulants, digoxin, thyroxine and iron preparations. It is likely that many other drugs may be bound by cholestyramine and it is therefore wise to administer cholestyramine 1 or 2 h after other drug therapy. The drug is contra-indicated in patients with intestinal malabsorption and in patients with severely deranged liver function because of the risk of hypoprothrombinaemia.

Prescribing Information

The adult dose is 4 g cholestyramine powder suspended in water administered 3–4 times daily before meals. Dosage may be adjusted according to response.

Cimetidine

See "Histamine H_2 Receptor Antagonists"

Codeine Phosphate

This is the cheapest opioid useful on the management of diarrhoea. In common with the other drugs of this group, it reduces intestinal motility and possibly also reduces intestinal secretion of fluid and electrolytes.

Pharmacokinetics

Codeine is well absorbed from the gastrointestinal tract and is eliminated by the liver with a half-life of 3–4 h.

Adverse Effects

Nausea and dizziness and constipation occur; otherwise codeine is free of serious adverse effects. There is little risk of addiction, but codeine may potentiate central nervous system depressant drugs.

Special Considerations

Codeine should be avoided in severe hepatic disease. The elderly are at risk of severe constipation and the very young may experience respiratory depression. Codeine should not be used in the irritable bowel syndrome and only with caution in ulcerative colitis.

Prescribing Information

Codeine phosphate may be given in doses of up to 60 mg three times a day to control diarrhoea, and patients should be advised to take the first dose of the day immediately upon waking to control urgency of defaecation.

Corticosteroids

Corticosteroids are used in pharmacological doses for their anti-inflammatory action for the treatment of some forms of hepatitis (Chap. 8) and in the treatment of inflammatory bowel disease (Chap. 5). The drug favoured for oral administration is prednisolone because it has potent anti-inflammatory action and unlike prednisone does not require metabolism in the liver to its active moiety. This is particularly important where hepatic disease is present and drug metabolism is therefore suspect. In the treatment of the acute emergency such as toxic dilatation in ulcerative colitis, parenteral administration of hydrocortisone is suitable.

Pharmacokinetics

Corticosteroids are eliminated by hepatic metabolism. The half-life of prednisolone is approximately 3 h and that of hydrocortisone, 1.5–2 h. Both are extensively bound to plasma proteins.

Adverse Effects

No significant adverse effects are associated with the acute administration of large doses of corticosteroids so that the drug should not be withheld in life-threatening situations. Continued administration of corticosteroids is associated with severe and occasionally catastrophic effects on the body. For this reason maintenance doses should always be at the lowest possible level to suppress the disease manifestations. Where possible, topical application of corticosteroids has the advantage of reducing systemic effects, e.g. prednisolone-containing enemata in the treatment of proctitis. The dose at which the adverse systemic effects of steroids appear varies between individuals. In general, a daily dose of prednisolone equivalent to 10 mg or below is not usually associated with dangerous complications. The adverse effects of steroids may be classified as follows:

Excessive glucocorticoid effect: Protein catabolism and increased gluconeogenesis lead to development of diabetes or loss of diabetic control, osteoporosis and vertebral collapse, myopathy, skin atrophy with bruising and striae, and poor healing. The effect on lipid metabolism leads to central redistribution of subcutaneous fat, giving rise to moon-face and buffalo hump appearances.

Excessive mineralocorticoid effect: Excessive administration of mineralocorticoids leads to salt and water retention and potassium wasting; thus cardiac failure and other oedematous conditions may be exacerbated, and in gastroenterological practice hypoproteinaemia due to hepatic disease, poor nutrition or protein losing enteropathy makes this side-effect particularly liable to occur. Hypertension may develop and glaucoma may be worsened. Potassium wasting leads to muscle weakness and may be profound in the presence of diarrhoea.

Excessive anti-inflammatory effect: The inflammatory response provides an important host defence mechanism and this mechanism is suppressed by corticosteroids. This may lead to poor healing of surgical wounds, development of peptic ulceration, predisposition to infection and masking of physical signs. The latter is of particular importance in gastroenterology as patients may perforate viscera without developing the usual signs of peritonitis.

Suppression of the pituitary/adrenal axis: Prolonged administration of pharmacological doses of corticosteroids leads to atrophy of the adrenal cortex and failure of the pituitary gland to secrete ACTH. In situations of stress or if the drug is abruptly withdrawn or stopped, dangerous hypocorticism may develop. All patients on regular steroid dosage should carry a steroid treatment card and should receive an increased corticosteroid dosage during periods of stress.

Miscellaneous: Various psychological abnormalities have been reported, ranging from depression or euphoria to frank psychoses. Cataracts may also develop, particularly in the elderly.

Special Considerations

The elimination of corticosteroids is enhanced by enzyme-inducing agents. In patients receiving these agents, such as epileptics, it may be necessary to double the dose of corticosteroid to achieve a therapeutic response. Patients with hepatic disease may be particularly liable to the long-term adverse effects of corticosteroids because hypoalbuminaemia results in decreased protein binding of prednisolone and there may be reduced hepatic elimination. Patients with hypoalbuminaemia readily develop oedema and patients with diarrhoea may develop profound hypokalaemia. Due to the inflammatory effects of corticosteroids the symptoms of peptic ulceration and even perforation may be masked. Diagnosis of intra-abdominal catastrophe is therefore more difficult. The elderly are particularly susceptible to steroid-induced osteoporosis and cardiac failure.

Prescribing Information

The starting dose of prednisolone for severe systemic illness should be approximately 60 mg per day in divided doses. This dose should be rapidly reduced depending upon response. The aim should be to achieve a maintenance dose below 10 mg per day. Once this dose is achieved it is advisable to reduce dosage very slowly, i.e. a reduction in daily dosage of 1–2 mg every month. When parenteral administration of steroids is required, hydrocortisone 100 mg every 4 h should be given by intravenous injection. Topical use of prednisolone may be achieved in proctitis by the twice daily administration of retention enemata. This therapy is of no use for more proximal colitis.

Diphenoxylate

Diphenoxylate is a synthetic analogue of pethidine used exclusively for control of diarrhoea. This therapeutic effect is attributable to its morphine-like properties within the gastrointestinal tract. In common with morphine, diphenoxylate decreases propulsive contractions within the small intestine and colon whilst at the same time increasing intraluminal pressure and causing non-propulsive smooth muscle spasms.

Pharmacokinetics

Diphenoxylate is rapidly absorbed, achieving peak levels at 2 h. It is metabolised by de-esterification to the active metabolite diphenoxilic acid. Elimination half-life is approximately 2.5 h.

Adverse Effects

The adverse effects of this drug are mainly related to its effect in slowing intestinal motility. Overdosage results in classical narcotic poisoning with respiratory depression, hypotension and coma. Naloxone is an effective antidote. Diphenoxylate is not abused. It is available only in the commercial product, Lomotil, which also contains a subtherapeutic amount of atropine. It is possible that the atropine discourages abuse of the drug.

Special considerations

Care should be exercised in any situation where constipating agents should be avoided, such as acute exacerbations of inflammatory bowel disease and chronic liver disease.

Prescribing Information

The drug is available as Lomotil, which contains 2.5 mg diphenoxylate and 0.025 mg atropine. Recommended adult dose is two tablets four times a day for as long as is necessary.

Disodium Cromoglycate

Whilst this drug has an important place in the therapy of bronchial asthma, its usefulness in the treatment of ulcerative colitis, for which it is promoted, is extremely limited (see Chap. 5). Initial studies produced encouraging reports of improvement in symptoms and histology in patients with mild proctitis. However, subsequent studies have been most disappointing. It has been proposed that in ulcerative colitis and proctitis, release of histamine and other autacoids from the rectal mucosa may be responsible for the inflammatory and ulcerative reaction. Because it is known that disodium cromoglycate stabilises mast cells against type I hypersensitivity reactions in bronchi, it was hoped that a similar effect might provide a therapeutic role for the drug in ulcerative colitis.

Pharmacokinetics

The drug is not absorbed after oral administration to any appreciable extent and is virtually completely non-toxic.

Prescribing Information

The recommended adult dose is 200 mg four times daily before meals.

Histamine H$_2$ Receptor Antagonists

This group of compounds is used in the treatment of reflux oesophagitis and gastric and duodenal ulceration, and may have a place in the therapy of bleeding gastric erosion and bleeding oesophageal varices. Blockade of the H$_2$ receptor results in suppression of basal acid output as well as inhibition of acid output in response to various stimulants, including histamine, pentagastrin, insulin and feeding. It appears to have no effect on sphincter pressure, gastric emptying or gastric secretion of pepsin and intrinsic factor. Changes in gastric mucus have been reported but their significance is as yet unknown. Two drugs are currently available in the United Kingdom, cimetidine and ranitidine. For discussion of their use, see Chaps. 1 and 2. It is likely that differences in the drugs are of only minor significance and these are evident from the notes below.

Cimetidine

Pharmacokinetics

Oral bioavailability is approximately 70%–90%. Peak plasma concentrations are achieved 60–90 min after administration and depend upon the rate of gastric emptying. Elimination half-life is approximately 2 h and cimetidine is mainly excreted unchanged in the urine. A small proportion of the drug is metabolised in the liver and undergoes enterohepatic recycling. The proportion metabolised increases as the dose increases. Plasma protein binding is insignificant.

Adverse Effects

These are infrequent and rarely troublesome. Gynaecomastia has been reported and it has been shown that prolactin levels increase after intravenous administration. Mental confusion occasionally occurs in the elderly and in patients with hepatic or renal failure. Transient and insignificant rises in serum creatinine and transaminases have been reported. It has been suggested that the hypochlorhydria produced by cimetidine could result in production of carcinogenic nitrosamine from bacteria in the stomach and it has been pointed out that cimetidine itself could be broken down to a potential carcinogen. The suggestion is at present theoretical with little evidence to back it up and the theory does not mitigate against the use of cimetidine in peptic ulcer disease. Cimetidine has been shown to reduce hepatic blood flow but the effect is probably transient and its clinical significance is uncertain.

Special Considerations

Cimetidine has been shown to inhibit hepatic microsomal enzymes. Inhibition of warfarin metabolism results in increased anticoagulant effect. It would be expected that other substrates for hepatic enzymes would be similarly affected;

thus levels of anticonvulsants, corticosteroids and theophylline may rise when administration of cimetidine is started. Patients with chronic renal failure may accumulate cimetidine and a 50% reduction in dose is advisable in severe renal failure. Caution should be exercised in patients with hepatic disease and in the elderly.

Prescribing Information

The usual adult dose is 200 mg three times a day and 400 mg at bedtime, for a period of 1 month or until the ulcer has healed. Subsequent therapy as 400 mg at night only appears to reduce the incidence of recurrence. Cimetidine may be given intravenously in a dose of 200 mg 4–6 hourly. Recent evidence suggests that a dose of 400 mg twice daily produces an adequate therapeutic response.

Ranitidine

Pharmacokinetics

This drug differs from cimetidine in having a bioavailability of approximately 50%. Less than 50% of the drug is excreted unchanged in the kidney after oral administration the remainder being eliminated by hepatic metabolism. There is significant presystemic metabolism. Protein binding is not significant. Elimination half-life is approximately 2 h.

Adverse Effects

Apart from minor biochemical changes similar to those of cimetidine, the drug seems free of side-effects. Gynaecomastia has only rarely been reported and the drug does not cause elevation of prolactin levels. Ranitidine has no effect on hepatic microsomal enzymes, but there is some evidence of reduced liver blood flow.

Special Precautions

Somewhat elevated blood levels of ranitidine occur in both renal failure and chronic liver disease, and the half-life is prolonged in the elderly. Adjustment of dosage should be considered under these circumstances.

Prescribing Information

The adult oral dose of ranitidine is 150 mg twice daily. Ranitidine may be given intravenously when the recommended dose is 50 mg.

Lactulose

This is a synthetic disaccharide which can be used as a laxative; its most important usage, however, is in the management of portosystemic encephalopathy (see

Chap. 8). In the latter condition it is more effective than other laxatives, such as magnesium hydroxide, given in doses to produce similar stool weight and frequency. Lactulose is not broken down by disaccharidase enzymes in the small intestine and passes unchanged into the colon. In the colon it is broken down by bacteria such as the *Lactobacillus* and *Streptococcus faecalis* to lactic acid and acetic acid. Stool osmolarity is increased and pH lowered. Free ammonia is ionised to ammonium ions which are less readily absorbed into the bloodstream. It is possible that this is the main action of lactulose in preventing hepatic encephalopathy, and the lowering of stool pH seems essential for it to lower blood ammonium levels. However, increased ammonium excretion has not been shown and the cathartic effect of lactulose undoubtedly contributes to its action. A reduction in urea producing micro-organisms and in other toxic products has been postulated.

Adverse Effects

Abdominal distension with colic, flatulence, nausea and vomiting are common in excessive dosage. Excessive fluid losses and hyponatraemia occur in patients with severe diarrhoea.

Special Considerations

Patients with galactosaemia should avoid the commercially available preparations which also contain galactose.

Prescribing Information

Lactulose is available in the commercial preparation Duphalac, which is a pale yellow syrup. Five millilitres contains 3.35 g lactulose, 0.3 g lactose and 0.55 g galactose. The dose for hepatic encephalopathy is initially 30–50 ml three times a day, and subsequently the dose is adjusted to produce two or three soft stools each day.

Loperamide

This relatively new anti-diarrhoeal agent has certain advantages over the older agents. There is evidence that it is more effective than codeine or diphenoxylate in controlling acute diarrhoea due to gastroenteritis, and the drug is of proven efficacy in chronic diarrhoea due to irritable bowel syndrome and inflammatory bowel disease (Chaps. 4–6). Loperamide is a piperidine derivative and slows gastrointestinal motility by an effect on both circular and longitudinal muscle of the intestine. It binds to opioid receptors and its action is at least in part explained by this mechanism. It is also claimed to have an effect on the cholinergic mechanisms in the gut. Large doses of loperamide are capable of suppressing withdrawal symptoms in opium-dependent animals. However, in man penetration into the central nervous system is very low; central nervous system depression does not therefore occur at therapeutic doses. The possibility of a morphine-like effect should, however, be borne in mind in patients taking accidental or suicidal overdosage.

Pharmacokinetics

The drug is incompletely absorbed from the gastrointestinal tract, and peak plasma levels are achieved about 4 h after ingestion. It is extensively bound to plasma proteins. Elimination is largely by hepatic metabolism and the half-life is between 7 and 14 h.

Adverse Effects

Headache, abdominal cramps and occasional skin rashes have been reported.

Special Considerations

In common with other anti-diarrhoeal agents, the drug should not be prescribed to patients with decompensated liver disease who are at risk of developing hepatic encephalopathy.

Prescribing Information

The adult dose of loperamide is 4 mg initially followed by 2 mg after each loose stool up to a total of 16 mg per day.

Mebeverine

This drug relaxes smooth muscle of the gastrointestinal tract and has been useful in the management of irritable bowel syndrome and oesophageal spasm in achalasia of the cardia (see Chaps. 1, 6). Unlike other drugs used for this purpose it has no anticholinergic activity. It is therefore relatively free of side-effects and there are no serious adverse reactions to the drug. Caution should, however, be exercised in patients with total ulcerative colitis as the drug may encourage the onset of toxic megacolon.

Prescribing Information

Dose of the drug for adults is 135 mg three times a day before meals.

Metoclopramide

This derivative of procainamide has been available for about 12 years. It has a unique pharmacological profile which makes it a highly effective anti-emetic. It has also been shown to give symptomatic relief in some patients with gastro-oesophageal reflux (see Chap. 1). However, the drug causes a number of serious adverse effects, and it should never be prescribed for trivial complaints. The drug's main actions are a central anti-dopaminergic effect, and a local effect within the gastrointestinal tract. Dopamine antagonism in the chemoreceptor trigger zone contributes to the drug's anti-emetic effect. An anti-dopaminergic effect in the basal ganglia accounts for the high incidence of extrapyramidal side-effects, and the effect in the hypothalamus causes hyperprolactinaemia in both sexes. In the gastrointestinal tract the drug causes an increased tone in the lower oesophageal sphincter. It promotes gastric contractions and gastric emptying and increases peristalsis in the small intestine. These effects are blocked by atropine. They are not accompanied by any effect on gastric or intestinal secretions. The rapid gastric emptying contributes to the drug's anti-emetic effect and this seems particularly applicable to the nausea associated with migraine in which gastric stasis occurs. The increased pressure of the lower oesophageal sphincter accounts for its potential use in patients with gastro-oesophageal reflux. Metoclopramide increases the speed of absorption of most drugs by rapidly delivering them to the small intestine and the drug has recently been incorporated with paracetamol to speed the latter's onset of action. However, in view of the drug's complex pharmacological actions and high incidence of adverse effects, such combinations seem inappropriate. The bioavailability of certain drugs is dependent on gastrointestinal motility; thus the levels of L-dopa, a drug which is partly destroyed in the stomach, are increased, whereas levels of digoxin, a poorly soluble agent, are decreased. The effects of metoclopramide on the gastrointestinal tract have also been utilised to improve barium studies.

Pharmacokinetics

The pharmacokinetics of metoclopramide are relatively understudied. It appears, however, to have an elimination half-life of 2–4 h in man and is not plasma protein bound. It is metabolised by the liver with significant first-pass effect.

Adverse Effects

Common side-effects include drowsiness and lassitude and occasionally bowel disturbances, dizziness and faintness. Because of the drug's actions, extrapyramidal reactions are quite common. Torticollis, facial spasms and oculogyric crises are sometimes seen at therapeutic dosages. The drug commonly causes galactorrhoea because of its effects on prolactin secretion. A history of metoclopramide ingestion should always be sought in patients presenting with this symptom. In overdosage, excitability and convulsions are common. They are best treated with intravenous diazepam rather than anticholinergic agents.

Special Considerations

Drug interactions through metoclopramide's action in the gastrointestinal tract should always be considered. Patients with chronic liver disease may metabolise the drug less well and are particularly susceptible to the central nervous system adverse effects. Patients with carcinoma of the breast should not receive the drug because of the stimulant effect of prolactin on breast tissue. Metoclopramide should not be used in the immediate postoperative period, after pyloroplasty or after gut anastomoses because of the stimulant effect on gut smooth muscle contraction. The drug should be avoided in the first trimester of pregnancy. The drug's effect in the gastrointestinal tract is blocked by anticholinergic drugs. Concurrent administration of major tranquillisers, especially phenothiazines, is considered ill advised.

Prescribing Information

The recommended adult dose of metoclopramide is 10 mg three times a day.

Metronidazole

Metronidazole, a nitroimidazole derivative, was first used in the treatment of trichomoniasis. Indications for its use are anaerobic bacterial infection, antibiotic-associated colitis (Chap. 2), intestinal and extraintestinal amoebic infection (Chap. 10), giardiasis and trichomoniasis.

Pharmacokinetics

The drug is rapidly absorbed after oral administration. Food delays absorption by an hour but has no effect on peak concentration or total absorption. The half-life varies between 6 and 11 h. Most of the drug is metabolised (hydroxylated and conjugated) in the liver and the metabolites excreted in urine. Accumulation may therefore occur in renal failure, though metabolism of metronidazole is little affected in cirrhosis or hepatosplenic schistosomiasis. It is minimally bound to plasma proteins. It is an inhibitor of various enzyme systems in the liver and consequently enhances the effect of warfarin and causes a disulfiram-type reaction with alcohol.

Adverse Effects

Gastrointestinal side-effects are the commonest: nausea, anorexia, diarrhoea, epigastric discomfort, abdominal colic and vomiting. An unpleasant metallic taste, furry tongue, glossitis and stomatitis also occur. Neurotoxic effects are: dizziness, vertigo, incoordination, ataxia and a partially reversible sensory neuropathy. Convulsions and encephalopathy have been noted on rare occasions; hence active CNS disease is considered a contra-indication. However, metronidazole has been used in hepatic encephalopathy without adverse effect. Other unusual side-effects are haematological (mild leucopenia and neutropenia), renal (urethritis, cystitis, darkening of urine due to a metabolite) and dermatological (urticaria, pruritus, rashes). Despite its tumour-inducing effects in animals, no such effect has been observed in man. Metronidazole should not be given in the first trimester of pregnancy.

Prescribing Information

Anaerobic infection: orally 400 mg three times daily; rectally 1 g three times daily for 3 days, then 1 g twice daily; intravenously 500 mg three times daily. All for up to 7 days. *Trichomoniasis*: orally 200 mg three times daily for 1 week, or 800 mg in the morning and 1.2 g at bedtime for 2 days. *Amoebiasis*: orally 800 mg three times daily for 5 or 10 days. *Giardiasis*: orally 2 g per day for 3 days.

Metronidazole is available as 200-mg and 400-mg tablets, 500-mg and 1-g suppositories, and 5 mg/ml infusion in bottles of 100 ml (500 mg). A suspension of benzoylmetronidazole 200 mg/5 ml is available for children.

Ranitidine

See "Histamine H_2 Receptor Antagonists"

Sulphasalazine

This drug is a compound of the antimicrobial sulphapyridine and salicylate. It is used in the long-term management of patients with inflammatory bowel disease, particularly ulcerative colitis (see Chap. 5). Although its exact mode of action is unknown, the therapeutic effect is clearly related to the salicylate portion of the molecule. Although sulphonamides and salicylates when given individually are absorbed in the small intestine, this chemical combination has to be broken down by colonic bacteria before substantial absorption can take place. It is therefore postulated that the combination of salicylate with sulphapyridine merely provides a vehicle for local release of anti-inflammatory salicylate in the colon. The concept is supported by the fact that rectally administered sulphasalazine, like aminosalicylic acid, is effective in improving ulcerative colitis whereas rectal sulphapyridine is useless. Several actions of sulphasalazine may be important. It has been shown to inhibit prostaglandin synthesis, to reduce secretion of salt and water into the colon and to reduce the colonic content of *E. coli* and *Clostridia*.

Pharmacokinetics

Approximately 30% of sulphasalazine is absorbed from the small intestine but the drug undergoes enterohepatic recirculation, either as parent drug or as an acetylated derivative. Absorbed sulphapyridine is acetylated within the liver, partly hydroxylated and glucuronidised. The elimination of the drug is therefore rate limited by hepatic acetylation and is consequently dependent on genetically determined acetylator status. Extensive colonic breakdown of sulphasalazine and slow acetylation both result in high plasma levels of sulphapyridine. Consequently high sulphapyridine plasma levels are associated with a good therapeutic response and a high instance of adverse effects, commonly in slow acetylators. The salicylate moiety of sulphasalazine is converted into 5-aminosalicylic acid. This is mainly excreted unchanged in the faeces although small amounts are absorbed and excreted in the urine.

Adverse Effects

Adverse effects with this drug are common. Gastrointestinal intolerance with nausea and vomiting may occur within the first few days of the drug's administration. This side-effect is dose related and commonly occurs in slow acetylators taking more than 4 g per day. Patients should not be denied the benefit of sulphasalazine treatment because of this adverse effect as the problem is usually overcome by restarting at a lower dose. Skin rashes may also occur early in drug therapy but are not an absolute contra-indication to restarting therapy at a lower dose once the reaction has subsided. Other forms of intolerance may also occur, for example headache and giddiness is widely reported. More serious adverse effects are associated with sulphasalazine therapy. Haematological abnormalities are particularly common. The drug may precipitate haemolytic anaemia in patients deficient of glucose-6-phosphate dehydrogenase and may also cause a cyanotic reaction in patients with congenital methaemaglobinaemia. Autoimmune haemolytic anaemia commonly occurs as well as irreversible agranulocytosis and thrombocytopenia. The drug has an anti-folic acid action which may manifest as a megaloblastic anaemia. Eosinophilia and fibrosing alveolitis have been reported. Raised transaminase levels, acute hepatic necrosis and granulomatous hepatitis have been seen. Most recently described of the catalogue of adverse effects is that of reversible azoospermia.

Special Considerations

Sulphasalazine chelates oral iron so that the two drugs should not be given concurrently. Sulphapyridine is highly bound to plasma proteins and may displace warfarin or oral hypoglycaemic agents. Patients with hepatic and renal disease are more likely to experience side-effects.

Prescribing Information

Sulphasalazine is available as 500-mg tablets; the usual dose is 1–2 g four times daily initially, reducing to a maintenance dose of 1.5–2.0 g per day. In the absence of adverse effects maintenance therapy should be indefinite in ulcerative colitis.

Ursodeoxycholic Acid

This bile salt derived from chenodeoxycholic acid is available for the medical treatment of gall-stones (see Chap. 7). It is similar in its pharmacological actions to chenodeoxycholic acid.

Adverse Effects

Although diarrhoea is occasionally reported, it is much less frequent than with chenodeoxycholic acid.

Special Considerations

Embryo toxicity has been observed in the rabbit so that ursodeoxycholic acid should only be used in women in whom pregnancy is prevented. Its use in the presence of gastric or duodenal ulcers is contra-indicated, nor should it be used in patients with severe acute or chronic liver disease, intra- or extrahepatic cholestasis, ileal resection or regional ileitis.

Prescribing Information

Ursodeoxycholic acid is available in the commercial preparation, Destolit, which is a plain white tablet containing 150 mg. The daily dose is three or four tablets according to body weight (approximately 8–10 mg/kg). The daily dose should be divided into two administrations after meals.

Drug Index

Subject Index